HOLLIS LANCE LIEBMAN

COMPLETE PHYSIQUE

YOUR ULTIMATE BODY TRANSFORMATION

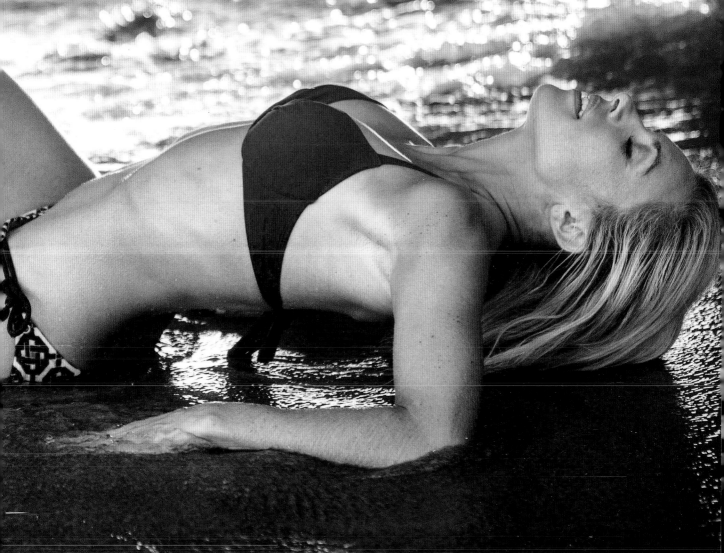

CONTENTS

COMPLETE PHYSIQUE

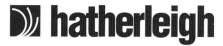

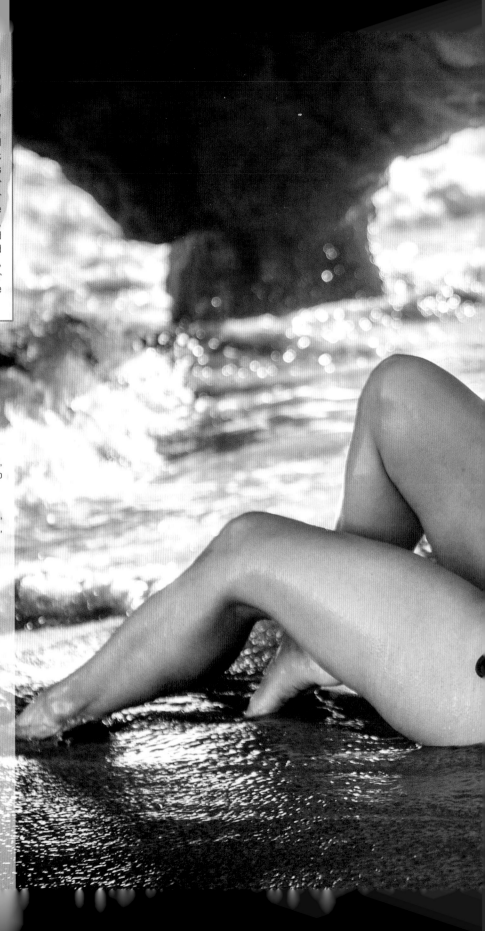

GENERAL DISCLAIMER

The contents of this book are intended to provide useful information to the general public. All materials, including texts, graphics, and images, are for informational purposes only and are not a substitute for medical diagnosis, advice, or treatment for specific medical conditions. All readers should seek expert medical care and consult their own physicians before commencing any exercise program or for any general or specific health issues. The author and publishers do not recommend or endorse specific treatments, procedures, advice, or other information found in this book and specifically disclaim all responsibility for any and all liability, loss, or risk, personal or otherwise, which is incurred as a consequence, directly or indirectly, of the use or application of any of the material in this publication.

Your health starts here! Workouts, nutrition, motivation, community...everything you need to build a better body from the inside out!

Visit us at www.getfitnow.com for videos, workouts, nutrition, recipes, community tips, and more!

COMPLETE PHYSIQUE

Library of Congress Cataloging-in-Publication Data is available.
ISBN: 978-1-57826-710-1

PHOTOGRAPHY by Jen Schmidt Photography
ART DIRECTION by Lisa Purcell
MODELS: Hollis Lance Liebman and Sarah Schreiber

Printed in the United States
10 9 8 7 6 5 4 3 2 1

》 hatherleigh

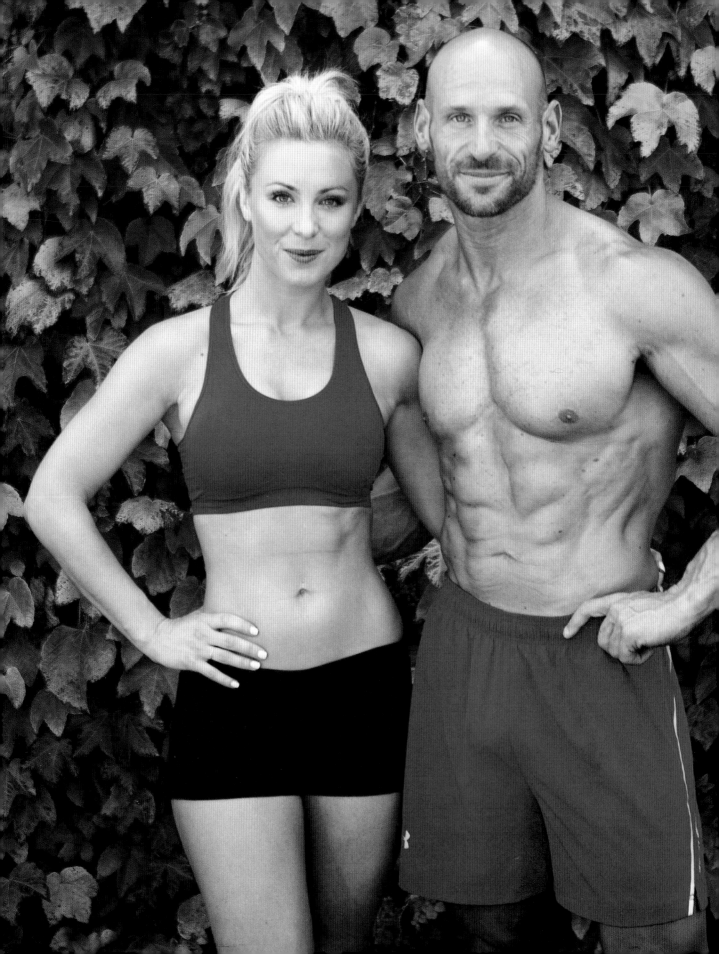

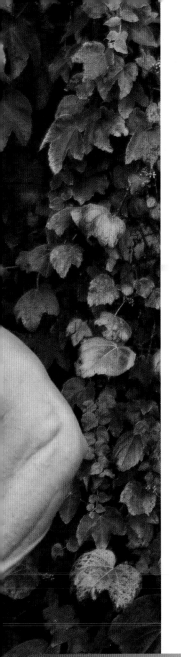

INTRODUCTION

THE JOURNEY COMMENCES

You are not alone. Not just in your sincere desire to get into shape, but in how you will actually get there. Now that you've picked up *Complete Physique*, you have every tool at your fingertips for bringing about the transformation to make *you* great again. This book is your story. It's not about who's lifting the most, who has more prominent abs or who looks best in a pair of pants or a dress, it's about you. It's about understanding that it's normal to feel self-conscious and intimidated in the gym and that the incremental victories such as your first pushup or pull-up more than make up for the pangs of insecurity that we all experience from time to time.

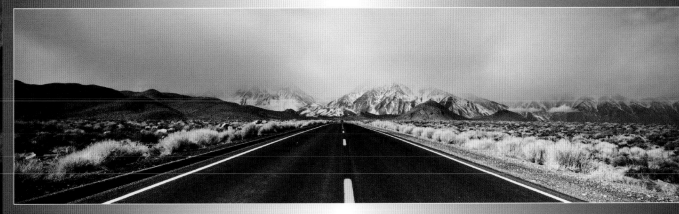

This book has been meticulously crafted for any lifestyle and/or starting point. It is my sincere hope that, from making this program your own, for life, you achieve the ultimate personal satisfaction of being pleased when you look in the mirror. This book doesn't just set you off on a temporary race, it guides you along in a continuing journey. There are, of course, moments when you will push harder, be a little stricter with your caloric intake in an attainable short-term effort to look good at the beach, fit into a wedding dress, or catch someone's eye at a reunion. But the *Complete Physique* program isn't about seeing how fast you can transform, but rather how transformative change can become permanence when the pedal is not floored, but rather steadily locked in cruise-control over the long haul.

The time to take action is now. No need to wait for a new year, another upcoming birthday or impending event, Your catalyst for change is simply *you*. Within these pages, you will be empowered to eat and work your way to a leaner and more powerful body without resorting to drastic measures for, at best, temporary results. You know that a salad and cardiovascular exercise alone is simply not going to work. It is the balanced program that yields balanced results.

A HIGHER PEAK

There is a man I saw for months at my gym. His face was drawn, his attitude serious and his efforts determined. He systematically whittled away week after week and month after month to hone his body to chiseled perfection. And then just like that, he stopped coming. Upon his return weeks later, he was noticeably heavier to the point that all the cuts in his muscles had been replaced by globs of shapeless, bloated fat. Why I pondered, would someone who clearly worked so hard, just give up his craftsmanship? Why this extreme rebound effect? Why would he sacrifice extreme effort and discipline to peak his body, only to seem less than complete?

For this book, I define the word complete not only as "all-encompassing" or "total," but also as "the sum of the most complementary parts," or quite simply, "You at your best." So with myriad fitness and nutrition books out there, why this one? Why *Complete Physique*? This book, told from the point of view of both author and practitioner, will keep you efficiently progressing from point A to point B so that you avoid the traps my fellow gym-goer described above fell into. This guide is gleaned from painstaking research and also from in the real-world trenches of application.

Let's be clear on why you're really here: you're looking to simultaneously lose body fat and gain lean muscle mass—the ultimate two-pronged goal. Let's also be clear on why you're not here: *Complete Physique* isn't about a achieving a finite state but instead it maps a targeted and systematic route that will take you to your destination, which is attaining your representational best. We are talking about long-term striking distance, but in order to get there, eventually, you must first reach an intermittent target. Just as a runner continues to run through the finish line and only slows down once the race is over and the time recorded, you can throttle back.

Most everyone is strong in pursuing their goals with regimented fortitude on Monday. This book will give you the tools to remain just as firm, focused and dedicated throughout the week. This book will reinforce what you already know: that you deserve to achieve your goals and in turn feel happy and proud of your accomplishments. This book will reinforce that living in a near-permanent rut, feeling sorry for yourself in a state that is both familiar and comfortable, need not be you. That the ever-slipping standards of excellence that many accept at being far less than their best need not be that state in which you live. Excellence, your excellence, is not only possible, it is essential.

NOT SUCH A FOUR-LETTER WORD

This is not a bodybuilding book. This is a self-building book that serves as my tailored guide to what truly works in getting you back to being your best, with timeless principles. The general public is neither concerned with nor interested in developing large muscles and putting them on display to be judged, but if you're reading this book, then you are concerned with losing body fat and showcasing lean and firm muscles, and that is, essentially, what a bodybuilder does.

Although experience dictates that stereotypes exist in any endeavor, and bodybuilding is certainly no exception, only a former competitive national champion bodybuilder (yours truly) is most familiar with the technical how-to aspects and the real-world experience of getting into peak shape. Sure, many nutritionists can get you skinny, but I have yet to see a client gain lean muscle while losing body fat over a period of time under the tutelage of said professional. The number

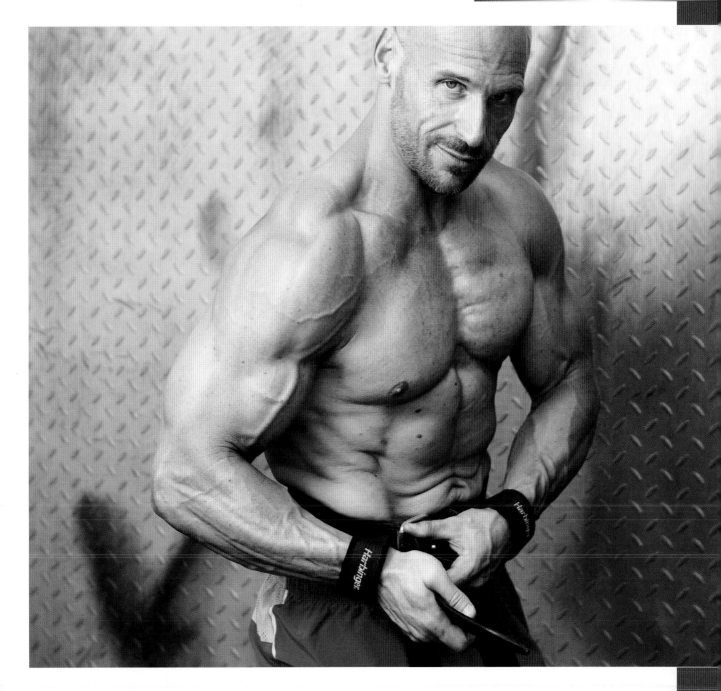

on the scale may go down, but the composition of that number doesn't improve. Ya hear me?

I'm proud of my bodybuilding past, and without the many years I endured under the cold steel, the endless chicken breasts I devoured at the dinner table, and all the posing I did under the hot lights in front of the scrutiny of the judges, this book would not be possible.

If you never thought you could, but wish you would, then this is the book for you. You don't need tedious hours in a gym daily, nor hours in the kitchen every day to produce the grandest of physiques. Whether you're a man or a woman, this is the Golden Fleece that we are all seeking, and within these pages is the map with which you will find it.

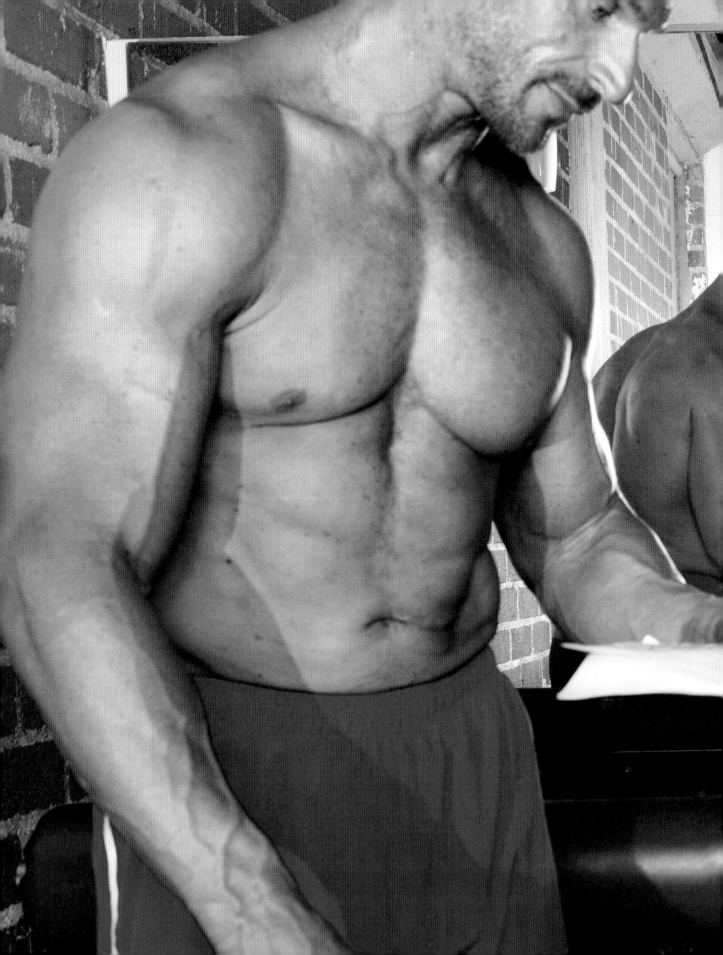

1 PLAN OVERVIEW

It's true that what worked once will often work again, but at what price? The law of diminishing returns says the longer and more one puts into something, the less one may take away, unless a variable is changed. The routine of any fitness and nutrition program allows boredom to creep in—and with boredom comes loss of motivation. What once seemed cutting edge feels more Groundhog Day with each passing repetition and spoonful. The cure is to find ways to keep things fresh.

...re, for increasing quality muscle development, a few exercises and a third day of abdominals have been added. And you still have weekends off!

...olism for a more efficient fat-incinerating state.

...an additional day of cardio will have been

MONDAY	Back/abdominals/30-minute cardio
TUESDAY	Chest/biceps//30-minute cardio
WEDNESDAY	OFF
THURSDAY	Legs/abdominals/30-minute cardio
FRIDAY	Shoulders/triceps/abdominals/30-minute cardio
SATURDAY	OFF
SUNDAY	

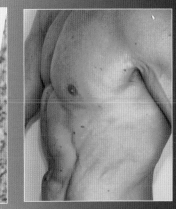

In my role as personal trainer, I see too many achieving too little in the way of results, and with too much effort. And as you know, achieving goals takes time, so give it time. I want you to stop switching gears every week or thinking doing more will bring about greater results. Different food delivery services, workouts, modalities and voluntary cosmetic surgeries, without giving any noticeable time to see if they actually work, will not bring you to the promised land. When I prepared for a photo shoot for this book, or in the past when I competed, I never reversed myself or questioned myself, I simply progressed, weekly. Give results, and ultimately yourself, a chance.

THE END COMPLETE

Complete Physique is a pivotal chapter in the ever-evolving story that is you. With its advancing exercises and routines, nutrition tips and motivation, at its heart, this book is the unabridged answer to the questions: "How do I maintain the spark, the motivation to keep going?" "How do I keep myself hungry so that I can keep moving ahead?" Or simply put, "How do I better myself?"

A major impetus for creating this book was my desire to address a very real and common concern that a friend shared with me. She said, "I am okay with being 60 pounds down. But give me a way to figure out how to stay here. Help me stop the cycle of creeping up and then forcing it back down, ad nauseam." Look no further, because the answer to that—and more—is all in here.

To begin your journey you need a catalyst to get you going. The catalyst for change is the need, followed by a plan and then acting on it. But progress occurs from a combination of things. When we become remotivated and reinvigorated, we are able to take things to a new level. After the photography for past projects was concluded, I continued training, but didn't quite floor the pedal so hard. I didn't eat as clean. I wasn't as meticulous about preparation, and so I gained some body fat, all the while remaining in somewhat striking distance of what I had previously achieved. But I hadn't kept the pedal to the floor because doing so simply wasn't feasible or realistic. Nor is it for anyone.

Later, when the need and urgency for this book occurred, I was again up for the challenge of embarking on my own journey and finding out the answer to the self-imposed question, "Could I be in even better shape for *Complete Physique?*"

As surely as there is always an X to mark the spot, once that X is crossed out, a new one appears. All of us from time to time slip off the track. Just as sensors in a modern car warn of a loss of air pressure in a tire, there are indicators within the human body to tell us that an adjustment is necessary. This book is your all-in-one resource to not only inflate and top off your tires, but to get them to perform better than ever. How good can you be? Let's find out.

PROGRAM BREAKDOWN

Complete Physique departs from the somewhat familiar structure of other fitness books. The difference, or upgrade if you will, is that here we expand the universe of exercises and angles, focusing on working with a training partner. It also features a complete portable workout (when short on time, location and/or training equipment), in addition to so much more. *Complete Physique* is gleaned from a lifetime of knowledge and experience that leads to real-world personalized results and relies on teamwork; ultimately delivering outstanding results in minimal time. Partner stretching has been included, as well as tips on how to properly spot your partner, yielding a truly complementary relationship. For the legions now living a plant-based lifestyle, a vegan menu has been added to include you into the realm of results with your carnivorous brethren.

The cornerstone of this book is that better is always better, not the standard "more is better" approach. It takes you through a 12-week transformational program that is divided into three progressive phases that each last four weeks. As you advance through each phase, you will see yourself become leaner, stronger and more muscular.

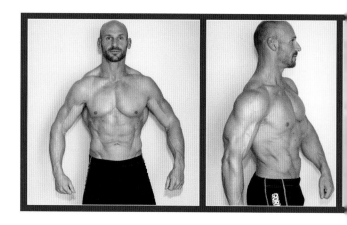

Whether you have a fundamental understanding of sequencing and firing from the correct muscles or are brand new to the world of resistance training and body transformation, you can dive right into the *Complete Physique* plan because cues and tips have been strategically placed throughout the program. Phase 1 starts you out on four days of weight training, with the maximum found in Phases 2 and 3. Phase 3 calls for additional and sometimes more advanced exercises. The extra effort has payoffs—again we are after long-term, noticeable results in minimal time.

PICTURE THIS

Forget about the scale, which at best provides a gross number, if you will, but not a net number. The first step is to take or have someone take pictures of you from all four sides, wearing a minimum of attire to attest to your true condition. Don't aim for flattering pictures: these will serve as your "before" progression indicators. When you compare them to the "after" photos you will take at week 12, the transformation will astonish you, telling a far more complete story than the numbers on a scale. I like to further instruct my clients to think sad, negative thoughts in the before pictures, making for a more dramatic after effect and progression.

The before-and-after pictures can attest to an amazing journey. When I had a client's 12-week progress pics blown up to a poster size to be revealed at one of my book signings, even he was astonished, let alone the audience. And it's moments such as these that truly define what the *Complete Physique* plan is all about. Remember that in life, our bodies are one of the few things that we have control over. All you have to do is truly believe this, and the world is yours.

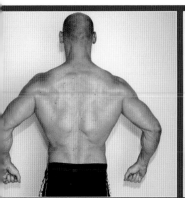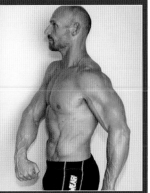

PROGRAM BREAKDOWN

PHASE 1: WEEKS 1–4
BEGINNER TRAINING PROTOCOL

Start off with a four-day-per-week body-part training split with three days of cardio and two days of direct abdominal work. You get three complete days off from exercise, making each "on" day really count. The key is to make it a habit—an actual lifestyle. Be sure to fire from the correct muscles. For example, when performing a pulldown, pull from the lats, keeping the biceps and forearms out of the movement. Place and keep the most tension on the targeted muscle without recruiting ancillary help.

MONDAY	Back/abdominals/30-minute cardio
TUESDAY	Chest/biceps
WEDNESDAY	OFF
THURSDAY	Legs/30-minute cardio
FRIDAY	Shoulders/triceps/abdominals/30-minute cardio
SATURDAY	OFF
SUNDAY	OFF

PHASE 2: WEEKS 5–8
INTERMEDIATE TRAINING PROTOCOL

At the beginning of week 5, your body is already showing signs of change—and for good reason. You've not only been doing the work, you've been properly fueling yourself to do the work. Here, an additional day of cardio will further speed up your metabolism for a more efficient fat-incinerating state. Furthermore, for increasing quality muscle development, a few exercises and a third day of abdominals have been added. And you still have weekends off!

MONDAY	Back/abdominals/30-minute cardio
TUESDAY	Chest/biceps/30-minute cardio
WEDNESDAY	OFF
THURSDAY	Legs/abdominals/30-minute cardio
FRIDAY	Shoulders/triceps/abdominals/30-minute cardio
SATURDAY	OFF
SUNDAY	OFF

PHASE 3: WEEKS 9–12
ADVANCED TRAINING PROTOCOL

You've reached the final phase of transformation. Four days of resistance training per week is carried over from the initial phase, but you now tack on an extra day of cardio and up each day to 40 minutes. This extra cardio will result in one thing: the additional shedding of unwanted and stubborn stored body fat. For further overall conditioning, some kettlebell exercises are included. Phase 3 is the culmination of all your efforts!

MONDAY	Back/abdominals/40-minute cardio
TUESDAY	Chest/biceps/abdominals/40-minute cardio
WEDNESDAY	OFF
THURSDAY	Legs/abdominals/40-minute cardio
FRIDAY	Shoulders/triceps/abdominals/40-minute cardio
SATURDAY	40-minute cardio
SUNDAY	OFF

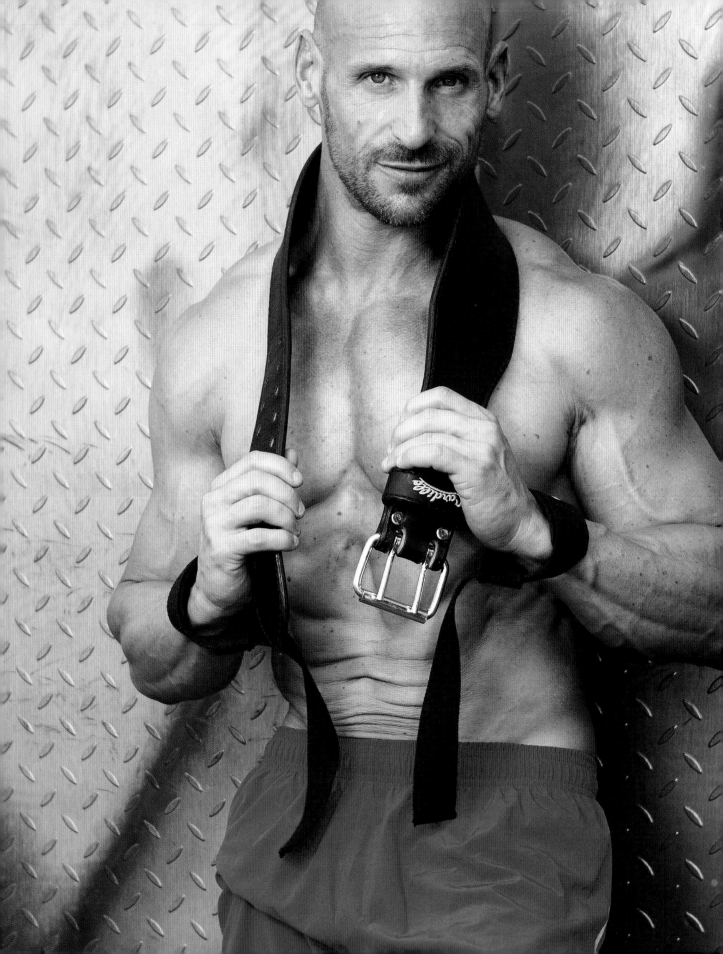

2 MYTHS DEBUNKED & TRUISMS

This chapter is designed to give you quick answers to burning questions and get you started almost immediately on your road to results. Myths are often half-truths at best and must be addressed, leaving no doubt in your mind that your transformation is possible and within your grasp. The goal here is to finish what you start (or at the least, show extreme progress), and the sooner you see results, the sooner you'll become a believer and life-long practitioner.

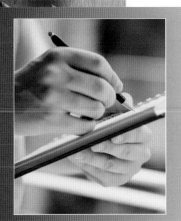
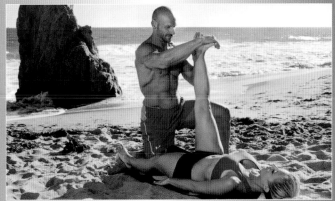
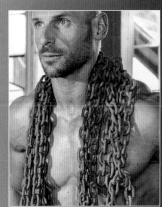

Q *Shouldn't I lose weight before I actually start weight training?*

A This approach seems logical enough. Lose weight and then build yourself back up, right? Real body change, however, starts with a change in perception. You should not be attempting to merely lose weight—your goal is to lose body fat and gain lean muscle mass. Just lowering the number on your scale generally turns you into a smaller, weaker, lethargic and mushier version of yourself. The more lean muscle mass you carry, the more calories you'll burn at rest and the faster and more efficient your metabolism will be. Resistance training, along with cardio and clean nutrition will result in the best you possible. Weights will both strengthen and firm your body, while cardio and proper nutrition will fuel you and reveal your body's true composition.

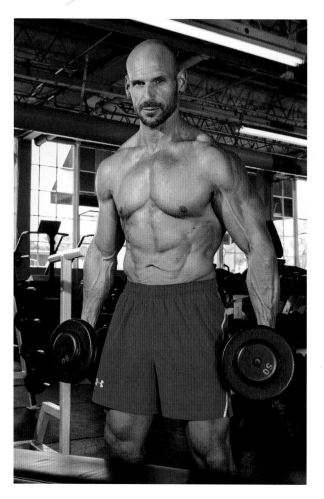

Q *I really don't enjoy lifting weights. Can't I just eat according to your plan and only do cardio?*

A You could, but you'd forfeit being a table that balances quite well on three legs, but now only has two. Not so sure if I'd trust it to be sturdy. This question stems more from a point of uncertainty. After all, you can just stroll into a gym and start up a cardio machine and proceed. But for those new to weight training, it can be intimidating to walk into a gym, this new world, and hoist the dumbbells. So often people stick to the familiar or safe. But I have yet to meet the person who performs regular resistance training and cardio and eats well who doesn't also love how his or her body looks and feels. I wrote this book and its predecessor with the newbie in mind. Within these pages you have the complete blueprint to resistance training and, when available, detail has been provided for giving you cues on how to properly fire from each muscle employed. The only thing not supplied here is the in-the-trenches, real-world experience that comes from spending time lifting weights in the gym. Remember, every champion had a Day 1.

Q *Why am I not leaning up? I'm eating mostly gluten-free, organic, vegan foods.*

A Recently, scores of consumers have migrated toward gluten-free, organic, no-meat, plant-based "diets." But until I read the word *unprocessed* on the labels of the foods these people are consuming, I remain skeptical. To replace meat-based products and offer the consumer a "healthier" alternative, food producers often add modified starches, GM (genetically modified) soybeans, artificial colorings, synthetic fortifiers, processed sugars, oils and other chemicals. In addition to all the processing, there often remains a surplus of fat and sugar hidden in these supposedly "clean" foods. If it is packaged and processed, be wary!

Q *Should I train on an empty stomach?*

A This is largely dependent upon your goals. A metabolism-boosting cardio session performed first thing in the morning on an empty stomach has proven to be highly effective for fat loss, dipping into stored adipose (fat) for fuel. For a lean muscle-building workout, it is imperative to consume fuel prior to exercise. You use stored carbohydrates in the form of glycogen to power resistance training, while you are attempting to dip into lipolysis (fat stores) to fuel cardiovascular activity. What isn't a good choice is performing intense cardio work while downing a shake or even eating food! In addition, perform your anaerobic work (resistance training) prior to cardio—flipping it the other way (cardio and then resistance) will only wear you out. And remember that the role of cardio is not to burn calories—which will be replaced as soon as you eat—but instead to elevate your metabolic rate and facilitate the assimilation of calories.

Q *Okay, I get it about eating something before the resistance portion of my workout, but I'm just not hungry, so how about something like an apple?*

A Sure, eat that apple, if your activity is perhaps typing, but there's very little energy in one apple and almost no protein. Having an apple or similar food before a workout is like going into battle with just a rock. You can always drink your calories when you're not hungry enough to chew real food. Protein shakes are an easy alternative to solid food; just be sure to include some fat with them, such as peanut butter, almond butter or chia seeds to slow down digestion and provide sustained energy throughout. And of course, always consume some form of protein with each meal, not only to help retain your muscle, but also to negate the release of insulin and the storage of body fat.

Q *I'll just drink straight alcohol and not add sugar.*

A And your hopes here are? Because rest assured that alcohol in whatever form is still seven empty calories per gram that will get stored as fat. Of course you need not give up drinking to achieve a complete physique. You need to be able to socialize, but don't feel embarrassed or peer pressured into indulging. If sipping club soda while your friends sip cocktails is not doing it for you, minimize the sugar intake by drinking less or having a drink with no added juice or heavy syrup or sweeteners.

For many, cutting out all alcohol is just too extreme. It would be tantamount to me cutting out my weekly cheat meal—and that would not work in the long-term. It's unrealistic for longer periods of time. So if you choose to drink, perhaps keep it to one or two meals per week. And, yes, wine, although it has some health benefits, is still high in sugar, an excess of which will bloat a physique.

Q *How do I avoid going to bed hungry?*

A I am not a fan of the practice that says "no carbs or eating after a certain time," for this will most likely lead to bingeing later that evening. I do believe and practice eating enough quality food to keep satiated but not overly full. You do not want to wake up in the middle of the night ravenous and overcome by temptation—you'll soon be raiding the fridge for a counterproductive midnight snack.

Including some fats and even complex carbs in your last meal of the day will help to keep you feeling satisfied and avoid going to bed hungry. Raw nuts, avocados, salmon or lean beef are excellent choices to include with dinner with lesser amounts of rice, beans or potatoes.

Q *Can you give me the real story on protein needs and exercise?*

A Protein in plain terms, is us. Protein is our flesh, our muscles. Everything else (fats and carbohydrates) is just energy. If your goal is to add lean muscle mass through resistance training, then getting enough protein is essential—perhaps even more essential than if you were pursuing other endurance sports, such as running or cycling, which are more reliant on energy (carbs and fats) and repetition.

For you to build muscle, you first need to fuel for resistance exercise and then go beyond what you have done before. For example, if your current best for the Dumbbell Upright Row is 15 pounds for six repetitions, then your goal for the next shoulder workout should be 15 pounds for seven repetitions.

You also need to include ample rest in order to improve. Protein is the fuel, the building block of growth, and is as important as training and recuperation to make the circle and process complete. Everything is working synergistically.

It is recommended to take in daily at least 1 gram of protein per pound of lean body weight and preferably even more. A 200-pound generally fit man should take in about 225 grams of protein per day in order to increase his lean muscle mass.

On a side note, provided the carbs you are consuming are low-glycemic, or low in sugar and insulin-releasing (more on this later), your fats are moderate and you are regularly performing cardio, you will become leaner, *not* bulked up as is often the common misconception.

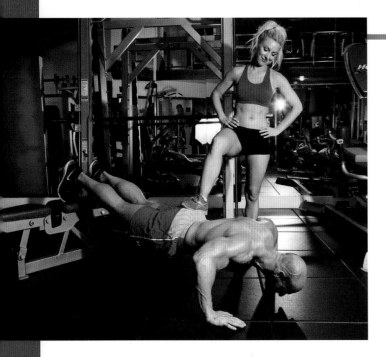

the next, works for you, that is fine, too. Just be sure that whichever cardio style you practice, it doesn't interfere with your weight training workouts and progressions (especially on leg day). Keep in mind the reason we perform cardio: it is to elevate your metabolism and burn more fat when you are at rest—it is not to burn calories (which are replaced at the next meal following your cardio workout).

Q *What's the difference between full-body workouts and body-part splits?*

A Both forms of workouts have their merits. Full-body workouts are good for overall conditioning and toning, as well as cardiovascular training. It forces the muscles to work cohesively. If you are short on time and can't get to a gym, a full-body workout, such as the Portable Workout (see chapter 7) is a good way to go.

Body-part split workouts (as this program is primarily designed for), are good for bringing greater development, detail and muscle control to individual body parts. You are also better able to train a particular muscle group to failure or exhaustion than in a full-body workout. The full-body workout may touch upon, say, legs, but only a true leg workout that is confined to just leg muscles will bring the most fatigue and, ultimately, the most lean mass to this complex musculature. For a more chiseled and honed look, the body-part split surpasses other modalities.

Q *Wouldn't yoga bring about the same results?*

A Yoga is a superb modality that has too many benefits to ignore, including flexibility and strength and improved posture, mood and circulation. Those who supplement weight training and cardio with yoga add diversity to their regimen. Although resistance training offers many of the same benefits as yoga, resistance training tends to build denser muscle than yoga alone will. This is largely due to the fact that yoga is reliant on your body weight, while resistance training allows you to employ nearly limitless amounts of weight.

Q *I can afford to either purchase equipment for my home or join a gym. Which should I choose?*

A There are so many affordable options for gym memberships today that nearly everyone interested in fitness can join one. For those

Q *I just saw an ad for this new supplement that simply melts away fat, and a friend recommended this piece of exercise equipment that practically does the work for you. What do you think?*

A There is no miracle exercise, no pill, powder or potion to rush your desired results, but it is indeed human nature to search for any and all such shortcuts and advantages. This book itself is the map, but you yourself must put in the legwork to look how you wish to look. There is no secret other than wanting it bad enough to do it and making it happen by consistency. Be wary of any such claims that you can get results by taking shortcuts. Although supplements themselves can help or simplify the process, the process still remains. In truth, spend more time practicing the solution rather than searching for a different way to ask the question—and then you will become the solution.

Q *Which is more effective for fat loss, sustained cardio or cardio interval training?*

A Either option makes a compelling argument. One school of thought proclaims that sustained cardio with less intensity preserves lean muscle mass; proponents of cardio interval training believe that it increases fat loss and provides a mental break from the previous monotony. For our purposes here, both schools of thought work. If you enjoy keeping a constant pace, go for sustained cardio. If alternating between a low intensity one minute and a higher who avoid gyms, it's sometimes not monetary limitations that keeps them out, but rather mental limitations. Some of us are just self-conscious working out in front of others. But keep in mind that the gym was designed for and will always be a place to better the self, not to put on a fashion show or to make others feel inferior. Years ago, I was at my local community gym as a newbie working out while my mother was in the hallway heading for the pool. As I was training, a fellow gym-goer made a comment to me about my mom's weight. He obviously didn't know that she was my mother, and although the comment hurt and I regret not telling him so, I learned a valuable lesson that day: never judge anyone in the gym, for they, like all of us, are there to better themselves.

When I train new clients, my job is to make them as comfortable as possible. I will generally collect some equipment and conduct the session in a corner, where they can get used to their surroundings and are less apt to feel quite so self-conscious. As time goes on and results follow, they are able to comfortably walk the floor with the best of them.

Of course, you can also work out privately at home or nearly anywhere. The main thing is that you work out somewhere. Still, I would almost always recommend joining a gym if you can afford it. Far too often training at home proves challenging because there are so many distractions. Often equipment that was initially purchased for home use winds up either alone in a corner full of dust, covered by some article of clothing, or on the block at the biannual garage sale. A gym affords you a multitude of options, and it can also offer boundless motivation and expert advice. After all, most people are at the gym for two reasons: to take a good selfie and to improve themselves. Get to it!

Q *What are the best exercises for isolating and toning the sagging part of my arms (triceps), muffin top (abdominals) and thighs (quadriceps)?*

A Spot reduction, targeting a very specific area of the body at the expense of others, simply does not work. The body draws fat as fuel from where it chooses. It is the muscles working together (compound exercises) that will tone more so than isolation exercises. Dip are far more effective than kickbacks for toning the triceps, and squats strengthen the quadriceps better than an inner/outer thigh machine will. As for the abdominals, clean eating (unprocessed whole foods), cardio and the stimulation received from your resistance training will always be more effective for defining your abs than crunches or sit-ups will ever hope to do.

Q *How do I avoid the "gym professors" when I'm in the middle of my workout?*

A I've spent the majority of my life in gyms, spanning different time zones, and in every one of them, I've never failed to spot (or be approached by) the person at the gym who seemingly knows it all (no one ever knows it all), and has a tip or two hundred for you. When I'm at the gym working out, I usually have my headphones on, which by itself is a good deterrent to mindless chitchat from others. I'm at the gym to better myself, not to make friends, pick up women or any other such activity. My advice is to go with your instincts and trust yourself and the process. If I see someone doing something with poor form or that is potentially harmful, I attempt to correct that person only after the set is completed, and then only in a respectful and helpful way—never in a talking-down tone. You could, in your quest for your complete physique, politely ward off uninvited intrusions. The good thing is that after some time, as you start progressing, you may find people coming up to you for answers to their questions.

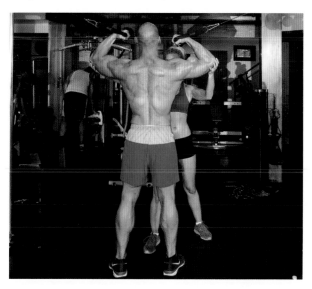

Q *What are some common mistakes that you see in the gym on a daily basis that might delay my progress or possibly even injure me?*

A The worst progress deterrent I routinely encounter at the gym is the desire to take on too much, too often and too soon. Less is more. Quality over quantity. Rather than strive to get the workout over with (which we all tend to do from time to time), fully commit to each workout, exercise and set and place tension on the targeted muscles.

Other specific errors are allowing the knee to go past the foot while squatting or lunging, wearing a weightlifting belt during the leg press and performing a behind-the-neck press or behind-the-neck pulldown rather than the proper versions to the front—all of these behaviors put you at risk of injury. Also, I see far too many gym-goers load way too much weight on machines, which allows them to perform only partial repetitions, especially on the leg press. The only thing this is strengthening is the ego. The negative, or stretched phase of a repetition, is actually the most critical point at which most of the micro-trauma is placed on your muscles. Avoiding a full range of motion is only limiting your ultimate best. Be strong, but be smart.

Q *Does it matter what time I work out?*

A It matters far less at what time you work out, than the fact that you are actually working out. Yet, the human body thrives on regularity. Some gym-goers wake up extra early and exercise prior to heading off to work, while others go after work. As long as you are properly fueled and able to get in a progressive and challenging workout, the time doesn't really matter.

Q *How many days straight can I work out before taking a break?*

A Again, the answer to this question comes down to your goals. For the *Complete Physique* plan, your main goal is fat loss coupled with gains in lean muscle mass. You most certainly could complete all your resistance training four days in a row without a break and still progress. But the key here is to stimulate, not annihilate. Rest periods have been strategically placed to allow you to repair your body and to be fresh for your next workout progression. It is for this reason that I like to perform a maximum of two days of strenuous resistance

training in a row and then rest my muscles on the third day. Cardio performed many days in succession is fine, but it should be performed at a relatively low intensity so that it will not interfere with the recuperation process. Remember, when it comes to your body and attaining your physique goals, *more* is not better, *better* is better!

Q *What can I do to make my resolutions really stick?*

A History tends to repeat itself. By early December of each year, with the holiday season in full swing, the masses set aside their physique goals or even maintenance. Come January, it's full steam ahead . . . for a few weeks, until those super lofty New Year's resolutions (like "I'm going to be in the gym every day and eat only egg whites and tuna") are deemed unreachable and thus abandoned. How do you avoid this trap? The first step is to pick an event or end date at which you are determined to look your best. The second step is to walk before you can run. Build intensity. Set small, incremental goals. Perhaps a certain poundage lifted on chest day, or to comfortably fit into a dress that was previously too tight. The third is to keep clean fuel on hand and a network of supporters in your corner. And the last step is to believe in yourself and be good to yourself. If you want a treat (here and there), have it—and then get right back on track. It's a cheat meal, not a cheat day.

Q *What are your real exercise philosophies? To look like you, don't you have to "take something"?*

A To look like me, one has to be born with certain genetic traits. For example, I have always been able to accrue muscle mass, but becoming lean has been the real challenge. Just as the pyramids were erected from sweat and stone, my body has been built over time using the same tools you will find within this book. What has built me is consistency (making fitness a lifestyle), placing tension on the targeted muscles when I exercise and steadily increasing my resistance, combined with clean food and ample recuperation. You absolutely can build an amazing physique equipped with the knowledge gleaned from within these pages. Consistency and commitment, regardless of genetics, will help you achieve your complete physique, just as it helped me achieve mine—and without the use of performance-enhancing substances.

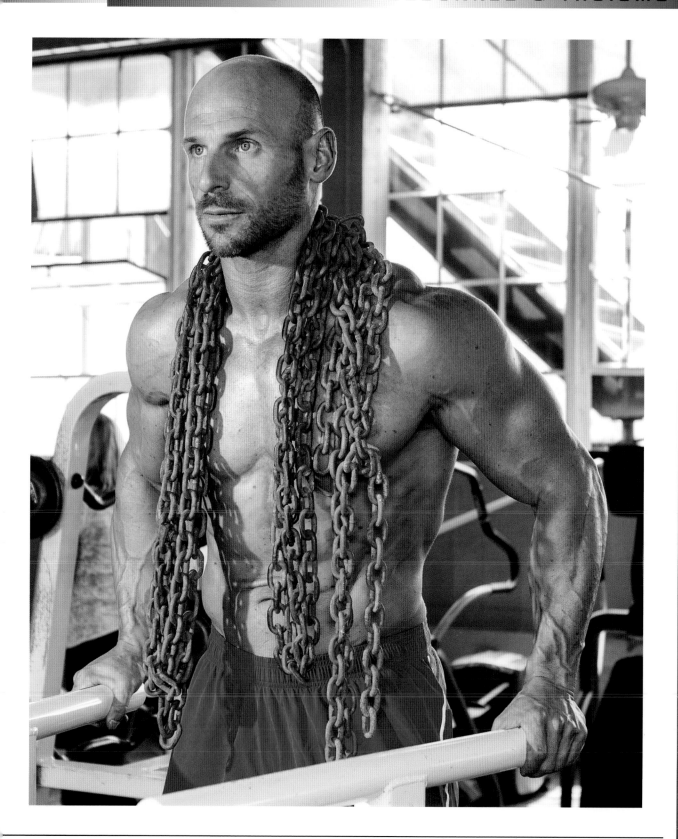

THE RULES OF YOUR TRANSFORMATION

For years I've been asked in my role as personal trainer, what I specialize in. My quick reply is usually, "I get people into shape." But that answer was really quite vague and didn't truly describe what I do, what I am undeniably passionate about and what my aim is to do for you. Please allow me to reintroduce myself: I specialize in transformation—your transformation. We're talking about pushing that giant reset button, getting you back to your best and telling you not just the what, but the why. For example, many books on your local store's shelves tell you the routines to do, but not the reason for the inclusion of particular exercises. In order to follow and excel at a lifestyle for the long-term, it's going to prove far more effective for you if you know why you are doing what you're doing. What follows are my top six key take-action items, which will make this your truest and most dramatic transformation, ever!

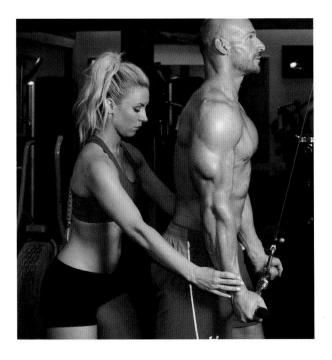

Employ the negative

Watch most people perform a pull-up, a push-up, a dip or even a curl, and you'll see that they often just cheat themselves. In an effort to claim they've lifted a heavier weight (or simply to get it over with), they fail to lower down all the way, at best, performing the belly, or strongest portion, of the movement.

The major issue here is that most of the micro-damage (a "good sore") caused by weight training occurs in the negative, or downward, portion of a lift, such as the descent in a squat. Failing to perform a full repetition results in less than full or optimum development. This is why one or two well placed swings from a hammer results in a well-driven nail when numerous half-hearted attempts rarely do.

It doesn't matter what the person next to you is lifting; it matters what the person in the mirror is lifting. Stretch and squeeze; by this, I mean get the greatest range of motion that you can. If you need to lower the weight in order to get a greater negative, do not hesitate to do so in order to increase your range of motion. Then when you perform the repetition, do so explosively, but with control. Resist the urge to just throw up the weight when performing the positive, or upward, portion of a curl, but take half a second to squeeze the biceps at the top of the movement to lock in the completion of the repetition and to also gain more control over the targeted muscles and avoid injury.

Spot

One of the key additions to this book is the introduction of a training partner and tips on proper spotting technique during the exercise breakdowns. A partner spotting you during your workout has multiple benefits; he or she provides you with both moral and physical support. A team is more capable than a single player. A good spotter will help you past the sticking point of an exercise and allow you to work beyond a point of temporary muscle failure. A capable spotter offers just enough assistance to allow you to finish the repetition, but not lift it for you.

For example, when performing the Smith Machine Flat Press, the spotter should be standing on the platform over the bar with a soft overhand grip offering light assistance when you reach the challenging part, usually at the halfway point before lockout. The spotter should not attempt to deadlift or curl the weight up with an underhand grip at the slightest hint that you are at a sticking point—this would take tension off your working muscles. A skilled spotter will allow you to still do the work, or the majority of it, and also enable you to get repetitions otherwise impossible due to the onset of temporary muscle failure. That ultimately equates to greater results. Think of a spotter as a skilled shoulder to cry on, there for consoling, while still allowing you to do most of the talking or, in this case, the lifting.

Progression

Progression: as in physically moving from one exercise to the next. Not in a fast or rushed manner, but in a tempered, consistent and fluid progression. You cannot rush through a routine to progress. You can rush to get injured, though. The program calls for a weekly investment of a maximum of four hours of your time resistance training, so don't hurry through it. Instead, take the energy you may feel yourself wanting to put into racing through your workout and put it into each and every set, making the most of your investments (sets) and your returns (muscular gains).

Set-up

Just as when giving a speech you firmly plant yourself in the middle of the front of the room before speaking, always set up an exercise properly before beginning it. Instead of grabbing a loaded barbell off the rack and diving right into an exercise, lift the bar from the rack, back up or find a space devoid of distractions. Then plant your feet and commence with the movement. If you're about to perform a set of Swiss Ball Wall Squats, get the ball firmly situated behind your lower back (your training partner can help you here), and square up your legs and feet before beginning your descent. Taking the time to properly set up everything will help to ensure smooth form, keep tension on the targeted muscles, allow you to get more out of each repetition, help to prevent any injuries and yield you the most from your time.

The right stuff

Working sets must be performed with the right muscles and with absolute integrity. If you're performing a set of Reverse Barbell Curls and swinging too much, you're using your lower-back muscles. That means it's time to lower the weight and use the right muscle—the biceps. The ego has no place in our endeavors here. Anyone can swing the weight up during, say, a Cable Lateral Raise, but keeping the body straight on and raising your arm directly out to the side, farthest from the joint, is a small detail that pays big dividends in the big picture: your "after" picture!

Journal

Keep a training journal, and update it regularly, honestly and effectively. You need not write down the workouts or every tiny detail, because they are here in this book. But recording your target sets—successful increases in lifts and repetitions over time—is imperative in order for you to progress. Otherwise, lift the same, look the same. In addition, target sets are most effective when utilized on multi-joint exercises rather than isolation exercises. For example, more muscles are worked and thus stimulated during a set of Front Squats than during Single-Leg Extensions because more muscles are actually working together during the former. This doesn't mean you shouldn't try to surpass your previous record for extensions, but your efforts would best be served focusing more on improving on your squat record.

Keeping a running and updated written log of your progressions will help to keep the guesswork out of your workouts and provide you with the knowledge of what you need to do to perform and, ultimately, improve. My gym journal always includes my target sets, the foods I eat or changes to my nutritional intake, my plans or goals that I am looking to reach and improve upon, and even any changes I am making in the weeks leading up to an event, be it a competition or a photo shoot.

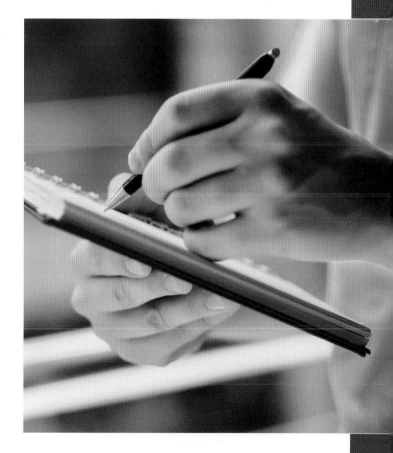

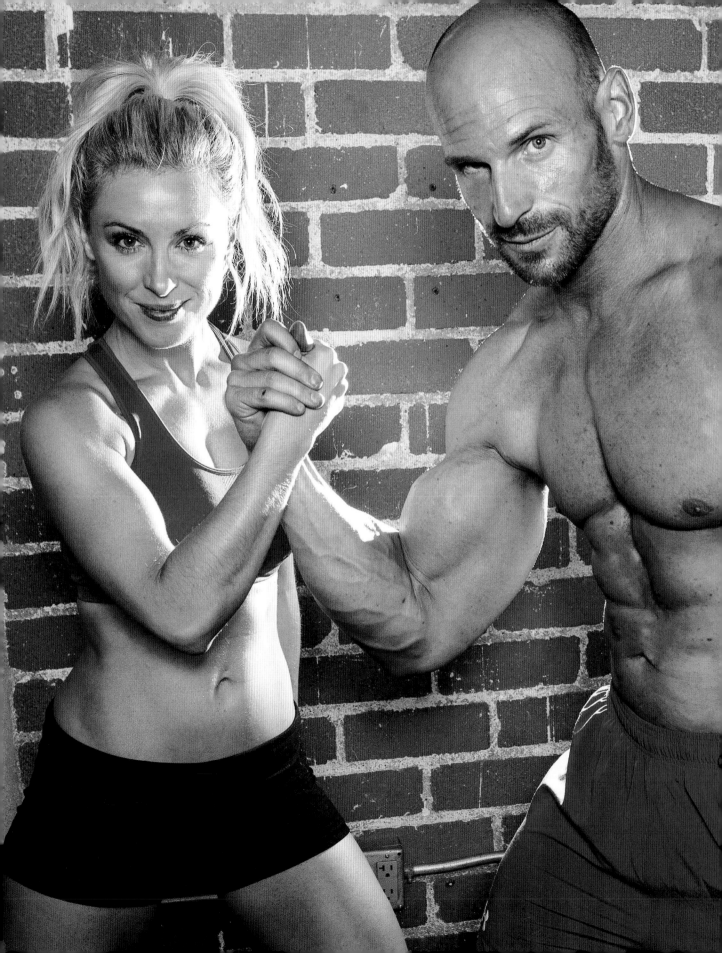

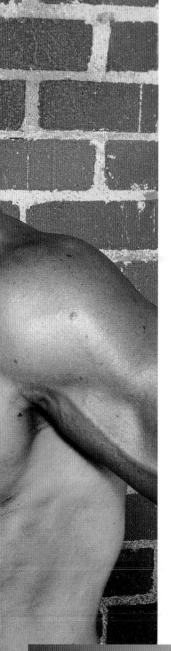

3 THE MENTAL EDGE

How many times have you set a goal, set a date for that goal, set aside time to achieve that goal and set aside time for that "last bit of fun" (in this case, gorging) before actually beginning that goal? We've all been there and decided after this one last binge, it's seriously going to be on like never before. But there's just one problem: "I'm going to" just doesn't work out, over the long term. You need to develop a mental edge that keeps your motivation sharp and the goal in sight.

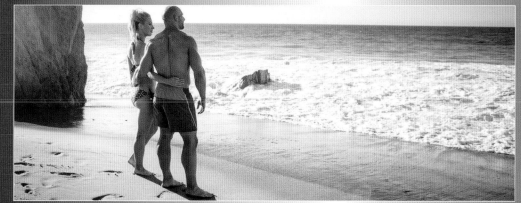
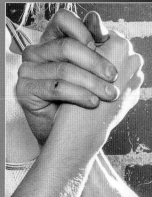

Many of us set unrealistic expectations when it comes to working out. We begin with excessive amounts of training and minimal amounts of nutrition and expect this "cramming" approach to yield magnificence. The reality is, in the end, it just isn't going to work.

Reaching a new level within yourself starts with clearly defining what the next step is, and the impetus to take that step is often derived from two simple, yet complex, mental acuities. What can you do to stay the course, and how can you avoid self-derailment? What is most important is that you work to become the kind of person who doesn't just say they will do a thing, but one who simply does it.

FORTIFYING THE SELF

Sometimes, as powerful as these means are—establishing an event to plan for, keeping clean fuel in the kitchen and maintaining progress pics to show positive transformation—they simply aren't enough. Sometimes, we need a little more to stay the course while also keeping sane about it. Sometimes, when you embark on a journey or take up arms in a private war that has you so in the zone, you lose sight of the big picture and why you are involved in the effort in the first place. And often more so the nearer you get to achieving that accomplishment.

In building and showcasing my own complete physique, I found that sometimes following the afore-mentioned tips or principles was simply not enough. Regularly posting my progress pics and positive catchphrases on social media was rewarding. Indeed, connecting with people is often a cure far more powerful than any other prescription. Surrounding yourself with like-minded, motivated companions will do wonders, ultimately lifting you from one plateau to another. We are all human and fallible and, as such, sometimes are enticed into give in to temptation. There were a few times while preparing myself for the photos within these pages that I wanted to give in. Yet the need to simply not give in was stronger than any temptation. And that need to stay the course was fortified when readers, fans and supporters let me know how inspirational I was to them during their own journeys. This in turn inspired me to keep on keeping on, when perhaps I would not have otherwise.

We can learn to redirect our minds, and this starts with passion. If we undertake something but lack passion, the results will be less than stellar. But if there is a clear need and strong desire to take action, then the results will never be in question—only the degree to which we achieve them. In other words, with this mind-set you will achieve a black belt master level in your chosen endeavor, the only question being to what degree.

When things seem to push a little too firmly against you on your journey, an unsupportive face attempts to steal your shine in a work or gym environment or even when the image in the mirror doesn't seem to smile back at you, that is the time for self-fortification. That is the time to truly have your own back and be good to yourself, because this is your journey, you're the one telling your story. Set your own standard and become who you want to become.

MY TOP 10 MENTAL ACTION ITEMS

What follows is my top 10 list of mental action items to keep you in check with yourself, motivated and progressing. Forget about what physically you feel you may not currently have—master these actions, and you will be prepared to make the changes you need.

1 If your interest or enthusiasm is waning, find the thread, or what you initially fell in love with, to get yourself back into the game. For *Complete Physique*, aside from sharing knowledge and helping you complete your journey, it was a personal goal to get into even better shape than I had for previous books. That was my catalyst to take action. I pulled out the calendar and circled the targeted photography date. I kept that date in mind, and it helped me get past days when I felt I wanted to give up.

2 Forget instant gratification and immediate pleasure. As experience shows us in before pictures, immediate results are not in the cards. In fact, the only immediacy about the *Complete Physique* plan is the immediate need to get started. Look not for instant gratification; focus on making each day your best through the powerful combination of effective training, proper fueling and adequate recuperation. Change might be slow to come, but it is most definitely progressive, and you can rest assured that if you're willing to invest in you, the results will yield large dividends.

3 If you're burning on fire (driven, passionate), offer to help light others, but never let them extinguish you. Not everyone is going to be supportive or happy for you, in anything you do. You be happy for you and also offer to lend a helping hand, without that needful hand ever bringing you down. It was quite something to see familiar faces in the gym—people who initially doubted me (I hadn't been in shape in years)—change their tune to, "Of course you're doing *Complete Physique* . . . you look incredible!" And as you achieve, your story further writes itself, draws people in and, in turn, gets others on your side and inspires them, too. The message is twofold: You can do anything if given the chance, and never let anyone limit what you will become.

4 Always keep your word, never let others limit what you may become, write your own destiny, and finish what you start. These are all big for me, a powerful four-pillar standing belief system in my mental arsenal. When you are gone, it won't be the ripped abs, hourglass figure or big arms that you'll be remembered for, but rather your word. If you say it, do it, and hold yourself accountable. Allow only yourself to define just how far you will go. You and you alone are running the show. All the way or none of the way. Start something, finish it. In keeping myself fortified and strong, I tend to keep my plans to myself, but share my actions with the world. Work in silence, achieve in the light. Only tell those you can trust your plans for you must self-fortify. Only when I've kept my mouth quiet and my actions loud, have things ever "happened" for me. Stay humble in character, but ferocious in seizing your dreams.

5 Consistency brings about results. Progress is not contingent upon marathon training sessions or a bland diet of egg whites and oatmeal. Extremes are not the heart of your transformation, but rather consistency in your entire approach. We're here for the long haul, baby.

6 Your body is ultimately what you do, not what you say you'll do. Are you a doer or a sayer? You can plan and read and study, but until you take action by really getting in the trenches, you're not transforming. Thinking up the solution may solve the equation on paper, but it does little to physically change it.

7 Chase your own shadow, not someone else's. We never have control over others, and we mustn't allow them to have power over us. This comes down to the human tendency to compare ourselves to other people. There's nothing wrong with comparing yourself to others if it motivates you or even spurs self-reflection. But putting yourself down or feeling inferior to someone else is a different matter entirely. When I was competing in bodybuilding, I never gave a care or worry to who my competition was for two reasons: I had no control over them and how they looked, and my competition was then, and remains now, only myself.

8 Here I quote professional wrestling legend and icon The Ultimate Warrior: "Ultimate Warrior embodies a kind of place you need to go if you want to get something done." That sums up how I felt for a long time. Something as life changing as a physique transformation is a daunting undertaking, and it takes a strong mind that is not easy to reverse to make it. For you to change, you must first deem yourself worthy and place yourself at the top of your list. To do that, you must believe as much in the mission as you do in yourself. You can fake intensity (for the short-term), but not passion—and passion is what gets you to your goals. My definition of "driven" is when you do the daily steps needed to achieve, even if no one else is watching.

9 Choose to live your life with a sense of urgency. Those armed with a reason are forced to take action and, ultimately, accomplish their goals. In movies, the protagonist draws us in, making us care by having a sense of urgency, by having a catalyst or cause that demands immediate action. You will reclaim your body and get into stellar shape by having the sense of urgency.

10 Perfection is not important because it is unachievable. Trying to live up to this perfect distorted image in your head of how you should look and lead your daily life is simply not attainable. Dramatic body change is not about any one thing done miraculously well, but rather daily actions consistently done well. No one lives a pure and perfect life. We all take a stumble sometimes. We all need a reset button from time to time. All of us. Yesterday is done and in the past. Focus on today. A change in one's body starts with an extreme determination, not extreme actions. And that change may indeed be imperfect because you are going to do it better and get better the further in you get. Forget the motto "Failure is not an option," and remember "To not even try is not an option."

DON'T DERAIL YOURSELF

You must hold onto the pulse of self-belief, and never allow others to take it from you or, even worse, give it away. Avoid self-defeating behaviors.

As you near your goals, often a voice in your head will complacently reassure you that "You've worked hard, you're there. Now's the time to coast." You can be assured that this voice is false and must be ignored. Coasting, and not complacency, comes after you reach your goals; you can't floor the pedal all the time.

Self-derailment comes at a variety of times and for a multitude of reasons. During my journey to get in shape for this book, I was generally motivated and staying on track Monday through Saturday. It was on the seventh day, the day of rest, that my mind would fill with unwelcome thoughts. Rather than fight them, or give in, I listened to what I was hearing, identifying the message behind them. By truly delving into what this self-defeating waste of energy was about, I narrowed down the main causes to a few key triggers: boredom, anxiety, loneliness, lack of variety and a deflated sense of ego. And I am speaking now not as a trainer, therapist or medical practitioner, but as your coach, the person to help you learn how to abandon self-defeat.

Let's take a closer look.

Problem: boredom: You may be happy to see all those OFFS in the Sunday row in the Program Breakdown, but with all of those days completely open with so much free time and nothing specific to focus on, you may find that your mind sometimes likes to create some sort of drama. Sometimes we either consciously or unconsciously create it to temporarily excite things and stir the pot.

For me, Sundays often filled me with the angst of choosing between scarfing down a certain pastrami sandwich or showcasing ripped abs. And this drama would begin with my imagining the "what ifs." What if I indulge in this meal right now in this state of instant gratification? That would be so pleasurable and amazing in the moment. And truth be told, an indulgence here and there is warranted, provided it neither negates your progress nor becomes a habit.

Solution: Find something else to be excited about, something that truly engages your mind. For me, Sundays became the day I flipped through fitness magazines, looking for inspiration for my photo shoot and getting excited about all the possibilities for it.

These hopeful thoughts let me forget about my possible derailment in the form of a mega cheat meal. What gets you excited?

Problem: anxiety: Generally speaking, that which we most fear happening, rarely happens—or at least it's seldom as bad as we fear. When pursuing a better body, maybe you dread being judged at the gym. My experience shows that others are simply too caught up in their own issues to give your worries a care. An example of this for me was at one of my book release/author signings. I was so nervous about how it would play out that I had trouble sleeping, obsessing about my performance at the event. Then a friend pointed out that as a fitness writer it wasn't my job to entertain or tell jokes but simply to provide good, solid fitness information to the attendees and supporters. And that was what I focused on, and I realized that every face in that room that day was a friendly one.

Solution: Face your anxieties and fears like you face everything else. What unresolved fear is holding you back?

Problem: deflated sense of ego: The truth is, our physical shape does indeed play a part in our mental self. How we view ourselves does stem, at least partially, from what the mirror and the scale reveals. You can't possibly feel good on the outside if you're feeling less than whole on the inside. I impress upon you again that your *Complete Physique* transformation is you vs. you. Often real change manifests from what is commonly known as the "black moment" in one's life. Commonly found in movies, this is when we find the protagonist to be at his or her lowest point. The good news is that the only direction from this point on is up.

Solution: Sometimes you need to reach that lowest point, or black moment, to truly rise. I implore you to hold on to this, to remember what brought you to this point in the first place. A big part of the fun truly is the journey. It's not only or entirely about the punch line (your after pictures). It's the gradual reveal of the joke (the process) that will serve you time and time again. You are more than worthy of becoming the changed you that you envision. What black moment caused you to take action?

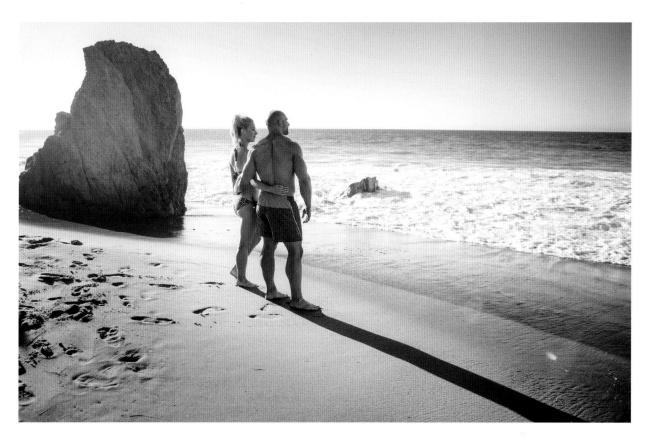

Problem: loneliness: Loneliness can often get one into trouble. I have always savored the incredible feeling of achievement that comes from getting goals accomplished on my own merits. Not having to depend on or rely on others has, for me, always paid great dividends. But the truth is, no one does it truly alone. Take this book, for example. I planned, wrote and modeled for it, but without the efforts of my talented editor and photographer, it would never have been completed.

Solution: Find and lock onto a pair of eyes that are taking the same journey—find training partners who will be nothing but supportive and understanding and who fight for the common cause. Who's got your back?

Problem: lack of variety: We need a plan we can live with. And a key to this is variety. Variety in the gym clothes we wear, the exercises we perform and, yes, the food that goes on our plate and in our stomachs. We lose our enthusiasm, otherwise.

Solution: Try out and pair new foods for a change that you can literally taste. Or perhaps ask a friend (with a strong fashion sense) just what works best for you. Find alternate exercises that target the muscles you need to work that day. What is one variable you can change that will renew your enthusiasm?

BACK OFF THE PEDAL

The *Complete Physique* plan is a time-specific program, yet designed so that you can easily live with it—and make it a way of life. It builds in intensity and complexity every 4 weeks for a total of 12. Doesn't sound like much, but three months is a vast amount of time in which to make an amazing transformation. Three months is also enough time to realize that you are running a well-metered marathon, not an all-out sprint. You are creating a sustainable lifestyle, not cramming a lifespan into 12 short weeks.

So, back off the pedal, but take your program seriously to make the most of it. Commit to 12 weeks and then ease off the intensity. Can you commit to prioritizing yourself for 12 weeks?

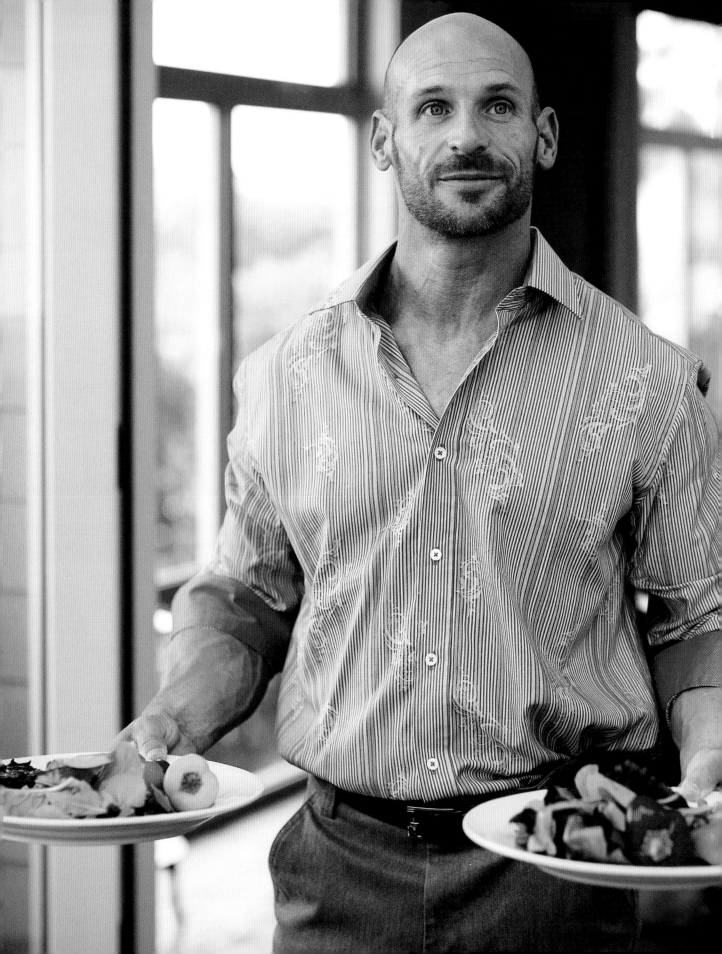

4
THE FUEL

If you follow a diet, you will ultimately and permanently fail. If you live a lifestyle you will consistently succeed. Read that again: Follow a diet, you fail. Live a lifestyle, you succeed.

Doctors, nutritionists and highly educated persons with plaques on their walls have written countless diet books, but as a former competitive bodybuilder, I know how to create a plan that maximizes lean muscle and minimizes body fat. I'm here to deliver it.

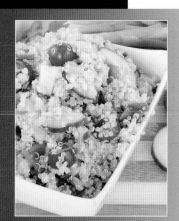
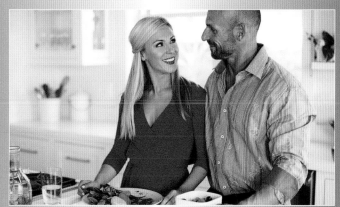
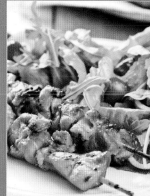

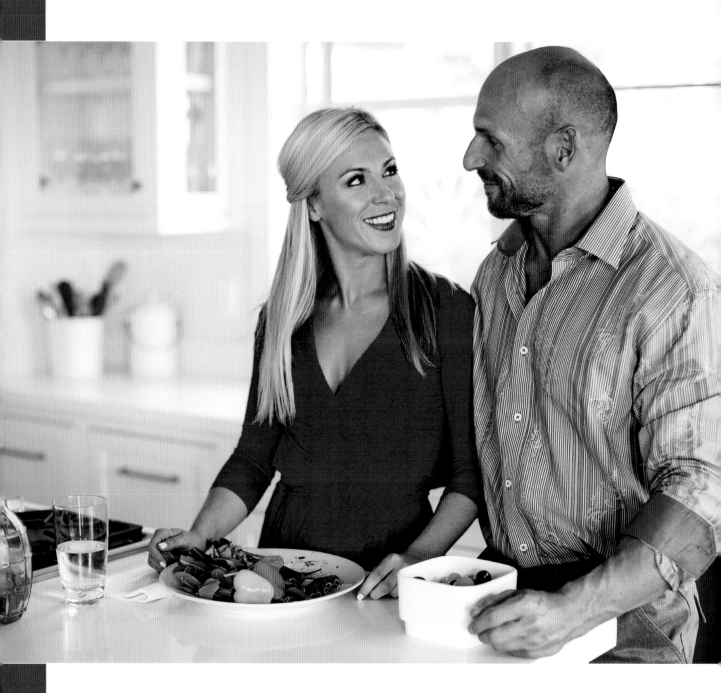

LEAVE THE DIET AT THE DOOR

Anyone can get skinny, but most weight-loss diets result in a drop in pounds that is, at best, temporary and comes with a price—usually muscle loss, which leaves you thin, often frail and soft to the touch. That's not what I'm here to deliver.

I long ago discarded traditional advice from nutritionists. Not that they have nothing to offer—they most certainly do—but my experience often proved the opposite of their teachings. One nutritionist insisted that all the "extra" protein in my diet was unnecessary . . . and she lost me right there. How else, I asked, do you hold onto muscle and lose body fat but by following a moderate-fat, moderate-carbohydrate, low-glycemic intake? When another suggested a very low-carbohydrate intake for many days on end, I concluded that what sometimes seems to work in a text book, doesn't work in the real world. When another teacher marked me wrong on a question asking which athlete needed more protein—the cyclist, gymnast, marathoner or bodybuilder—when I circled "bodybuilder" and was marked incorrect, I was done with traditional teachings.

If you thought of the body as akin to a house, you would be less concerned with its sheer square footage and more concerned with the quality of its framework. The *Complete Physique* fitness plan is not about dieting—it's about building a strong framework. That means coupling maximal lean muscle tissue with minimal body fat. Not enough attention is paid to paring those two things. It would seem to many that the two can't coexist, that it's seemingly just too difficult to achieve this balance. The many are absolutely wrong.

It also means banning the word *diet* from your vocabulary. Sure, it can just refer to the foods a person consumes, but these days the word comes with other baggage. The word *diet* now connotes "deprivation," in other words, depriving yourself to lose weight, often through unsustainable levels of food or unrealistic restrictions on your food choices. Replace the word *diet* with the word *intake*— a neutral term that harks back to diet's original meaning. It is simply what you eat.

CONSUME SMART

Consumers today know more than those of yesteryear. We know that even though a food product is labeled LOW FAT and LOW CALORIE, it's still very likely to be unhealthy—the reduction in fat and calories is the result of processing. Anything labeled with these words—unless you find them in the fresh veggie aisle—is a food product and is rarely raw or unrefined.

These days, we also know that a calorie is not just a calorie. Sure, anyone can shed pounds by reducing calorie intake—eating just about any foods—but the quality of the calories you consume ultimately plays a large role in your body's composition.

For example, which is better for you: a can of soda contains roughly 140 calories with 39 grams of sugar and 0 fiber or the equivalent 140 calories in raw nuts, with its 1 gram of sugar and 3 grams of dietary fiber? The clear choice is the raw nuts, because the soda is going to be stored as body fat.

Here's why: The soda will affect the body by bringing a sugar rush to the liver. To process this rush of sugar, the pancreas releases excessive amounts of insulin, which stores the sugar as fat. All this—even though soda contains no fat.

The raw nuts, on the other hand, do contain fat, and that fat, along with the nuts' fiber content, will digest much more slowly, maintaining blood sugar levels on a far more even keel. Another bonus is that the fat in the raw nuts will help to keep you satiated. A can of soda will just leave you hungry and craving even more sugar very soon thereafter. This is due to the fact that high insulin levels can block your brain from knowing that you are full, which can create powerful urges for more and more sugar.

NO FREE RIDE

No one gets a pass from sugar abuse and its ill effects. We often look at skinny people and assume that they must be healthy, but being thin isn't always the same as being healthy.

What are the "enviable" people eating? If they regularly consume processed foods, they might well be "skinny fat,"' and skinny-fat people can develop unhealthy fat around their organs. They may lack lean muscle, which can result in higher insulin resistance (the body's inability to use insulin effectively), and they might be at risk for developing diseases such as type 2 diabetes.

Fortunately, these negatives can be avoided if they lose body fat and exercise with resistance training to increase lean muscle mass, improve flexibility and develop true body composition health.

GET IT UNDER CONTROL

So what's the solution if you do carry extra weight? Why is it so hard to lose it? Contrary to popular opinion, obese persons were not born to be obese. Being "big-boned" or having "no metabolism" is a myth. Although a certain body type (endomorphic) has a predisposition to storing visible body fat and seemingly does so while simply looking at processed foods, the really good news is that even endomorphs have control over their bodies.

Even before portion control, try really "cleaning" up your food. This means choosing items to put in your shopping cart that generally reside at the outer perimeters of the supermarket: the vegetables and fruit, the meat and the dairy. The mid aisles generally contain processed foods, products that in the short term may seem cheaper, but are far more expensive in the long-term. Eating clean food equals a clean inner you and, ultimately, a clean outer you.

Remember that merely cutting back on processed foods is *still* eating processed foods. To become lean and stay healthy, stick with food that is consumed as close to its original state as possible.

EMOTIONAL EATING

Your transformation begins with identifying your triggers, those signs that you are heading toward nutritional derailment and eventually physique derailment. How to counteract a goal-thwarting behavior (cheating, binge eating) must be discussed before we can progress further. If the following behaviors apply to you, you may be an emotional eater:

- Do you begin Monday strong and in control, only to slide out of bounds and off the wagon Friday through Sunday? Do you then repeat the cycle come the next Monday?

- Do you often swear that after today, you'll drink not a single drop of alcohol ever, or that tomorrow you'll begin a very strict deprivation diet? When tomorrow comes and you see that the reality of your goal is at least a tad unrealistic, do you then abandon that goal?

- Do you make it through the day with both a proper workout and clean eating, only to seemingly purposely sabotage your efforts by vacuuming down junk only minutes before bedtime?

Why, for so many of us, is it all or nothing? Why do we set our sights on unrealistic goals that only set us up to fail? Do we really want to punish ourselves, to live with constant guilt? Why do we suddenly stuff our faces when dealing with a stressful situation in the hopes that this extreme will thwart another?

Emotional eating, which comes on rapidly, is using foods to make yourself feel better—although the only thing you really fill is your belly, not any emotional needs or gaps. Commonly referred to as "eating your feelings," this self-destructive behavior results in mindless overeating and leaves you feeling both physically and emotionally worse for wear. Like an addict who replaces something missing from life with drugs or alcohol, emotional eaters replace what's missing with food. That leaves emotional eaters walking a hard road. Unlike alcoholics and drug addicts, whose substance of choice isn't necessary for life, addictive eaters can't just give up food forever.

So what is that you are missing? What sends you to the refrigerator? Identifying these triggers is the first step in literally turning the scales in your favor. Boredom, frustration, stress, the need for instant gratification, anxiety, loneliness, exhaustion and,

yes, even the desire to celebrate with excessive food when happy, are all triggers that set off emotional eating. Feeling as if you have little to nothing to look forward to and an inability to tolerate your own bad feelings are also strong triggers for surrendering to emotional eating.

Emotional eating is a particularly destructive behavior because indulging becomes your primary coping mechanism in an unhealthy impulse cycle that leaves you feeling, at best, good in the moment but worse for wear over the long haul in a vicious and ongoing process. Of course, sometimes even knowing a certain behavior is bad isn't enough for you to stop doing it—it's not that difficult to find a reason or excuse for allowing such poor practice.

Perhaps you may find yourself believing that you had an especially tough day, a day of careful eating and strenuous training, and you indeed deserve this immediate gluttony. And let's face it, when you're eating the burger or pizza or whatever your favorite treat is, life couldn't be better. The short term "high" you receive from the flavors of your favorite foods exploding in your mouth can be extraordinary—in the short term. Yet, even the planning of an indulgence is part of the cycle of emotional eating.

Yet, the guilt associated with emotional eating is too great a burden to bear, too great an indulgence to dismiss, and it can't coexist with a social life. Some emotional eaters punish themselves with seclusion, even canceling events for fear of their "secret indulgence" behavior being discovered.

CONSCIOUS EATING

You must work to replace the mental confinement of emotional eating with the freedom of conscious eating. "Conscious eating" means that you eat when you feel physically hungry, which is a natural feeling. You then stop eating at the point of feeling satiated, but not overly full or stuffed. You are aware of what you are putting into your body.

Conscious eaters do not replace negative emotions with the temporary positive feeling associated with instant gratification and emotional eating. Conscious eaters plan ahead by packing food to bring with them to work, on the road and for any eventuality, and they further know how and what to order when placed in a situation in which they could just throw it all out the window and give into temptation. Conscious eaters do not allow themselves to get too hungry, which

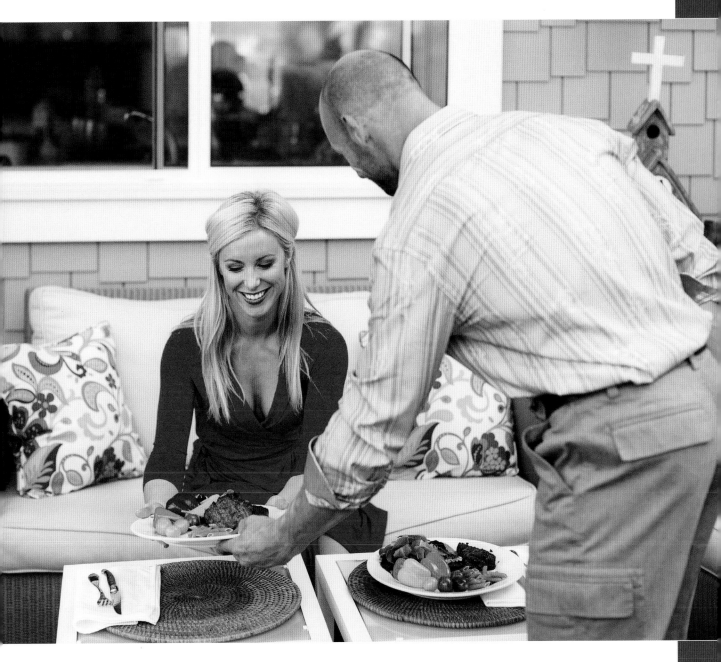

could create an emotional eating trigger, nor do they have negative relationships with their bodies or even food itself.

Just how can you protect and fortify yourself in your role as a conscious eater? Taking the time to prepare healthy food ahead of time is not only fueling you for optimal performance and aesthetics, but is also reaffirming that loving yourself is good and that your self-worth is high. You can further take back control and make the shift from emotional eating to conscious eating by slowing down, breathing, enjoying your food and never skipping meals. Find activities or passions that are positive, ones that leave you feeling happy and keep you in the moment. Cultivating healthy habits and supportive friends can go a long way to keeping you whole and in control of your lifestyle.

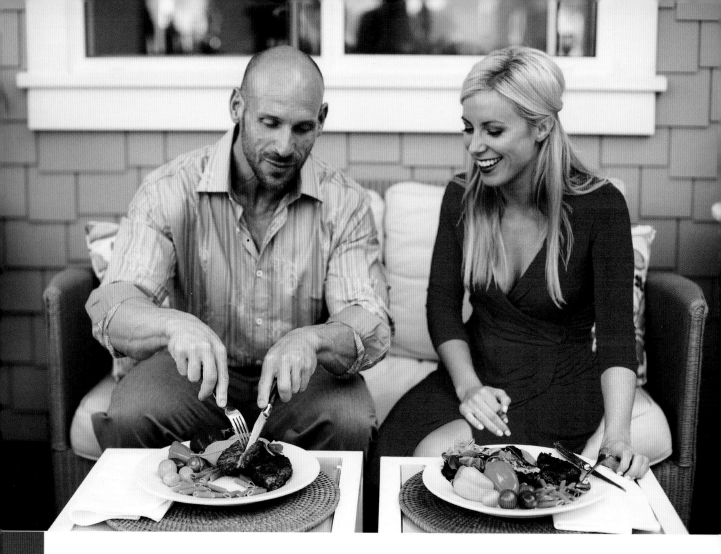

THE PEERS & THE PRESSURE

Recently, I took a date to a sushi restaurant. Not a problem, I thought. There's plenty of healthy choices. When my date asked me what I was ordering, she didn't seem too impressed with my selection. Too clean, I fathomed from her reaction. When I asked what she liked, there wasn't one choice that wasn't fried and bathed in a heavy sauce. She gave me the eyes and said, "You wouldn't let a girl eat by herself, would you?" And so although there was no gun put to my head, I indulged and had an unplanned cheat meal. Certainly not the biggest of blunders. But I felt a mixture of guilt and annoyance. Sound familiar?

Far too often we derail ourselves because our partner, loved one, friend or what have you is not on board. They judge. And we want to at least placate, to be liked, to fit in, to not rock the boat, to not be judged. But other people's choices should not impede your progress or negate your goals. The ones who get it are your peers. Keep them around you. Ignore the people

who pressure you, the people who thwart your efforts because they are unable or unwilling to follow the same path. Pay them no mind.

In life it's often important to compromise, but it's also important to have someone's back and to appreciate those who have yours. Be true to you. What I might have done differently on that date is never to have had it in the first place, because we didn't have another. Yet, in all seriousness, I could have explained to her that this is my lifestyle and the way I wish to eat. By all means order what you like. It's that simple.

If you're concerned with offending others, don't be. Once your body starts changing, it is you they will look up to for actually walking the walk. In truth, what is needed in life and in your pursuit of a complete physique is more "Did you eat meal 4?" and less "Why are you eating so many meals?" When in doubt, you eat the foods that you are comfortable eating, regardless of the company you are keeping. People tend to respect those who do not reverse themselves.

A DIFFERENT KIND OF PROCESS

Most of us have heard about portion control and warnings to not shop for food while hungry, and to some degree these are effective strategies, but I'm going to share with you some in-the-trenches solutions that continue to serve me well. We're all on the same page here: none of us want to get comfortable in "fat clothes," so let's thwart the pulverizing beast that is nutritional derailment by mastering the mental in order to enhance the physical.

Some of the measures I've used over the years to get myself into peak condition (or even in the realm of it) may seem humorous or a little outside the box (and indeed they are), but they work for me. The more strategies you can employ, the more fortified you become and better prepared to achieve your goals.

Gorging on food shows

If I can't eat it, I watch it. For me, watching someone else indulge while I can't has always had a powerfully positive effect—I'm living vicariously through them without the guilt. So if watching a TV show dedicated to searching the country for the greatest pig-out spot or getting hooked on cupcake competitions sates your appetite without sending you to the nearest barbecue joint or bakery, wallow in your favorite foods on screen.

Take 'em out

It sure is fun to watch someone eat sinfully good food and then ask them questions about it . . . a lot of questions, as I tend to do. Countless times have I taken out friends, relatives and even dates for a lavish meal and then deposed them like an attorney about every aspect of it. And they're usually good sports. My favorite question, asked just as a friend takes the first bite of a decadent treat, is: "Describe for me what's going on right now on your palate." The answers make those restaurant checks my favorite bills to pay.

Clothes shopping

There's two ways of looking at this activity: You either force yourself out of the baggy sweatpants and loose-fitting shorts to try more form-fitting and flattering attire that does not yet fit but ultimately will, or you can reward yourself by trying on clothes that fit now, ones that quite frankly make you feel and look fine. The former can work as incentive—think about how that dress is going to accentuate your new curves. The latter way can be a reward for your hard work up to that point. You don't have to settle for what many call a "fat wardrobe." When jeans fit and your waist is looking small, there's little chance of you allowing yourself to derail your efforts.

Photographs

Let's face it, if you're not feeling your best or even good, you probably won't want to take progress pictures. But I've always found that if a serious urge to indulge in a cheat meal strikes, and you're showing some progress, no matter how minute, snap some pics. Finding something to like about your body and even the tiniest hint of a smile will indeed help to keep you on track. And if you're really liking the pics, post 'em on social media.

Reach out on social media

When I was a competitive bodybuilder, we didn't have social media, but the immediacy associated with it is now such a part of our lives. Back then, I'd go into my buddy's office at the gym, strip down to my skivvies and hit some poses. If I was on track, he'd smile. If I wasn't, I'd get the look of disappointment. And that was that as far as feedback went. Today, posting progress pics does so much to keep you on track and to let you know that you are doing a good job and in turn inspiring others. Those "likes" and "comments" really do add to your arsenal. And surfing through others' social media accounts can be extremely motivational. It's impossible for me to scroll through people I am following and not be motivated to stay strong, keeping on my program and eating clean, when I see all their progress pics and positive phrases. Remember, those who inspire in turn need to be inspired themselves. We're all in this together!

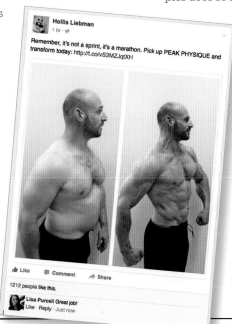

SWEET DANGER

Let's begin our talk about food intake openly and honestly and recognize the elephant in the room: sugar. Sugar, a simple carbohydrate generally used to sweeten foods and drinks and, more specifically, foods that are processed. Processed foods are altered from their natural state to offer convenience and flavor, but all that added sugar takes its toll. Consumption of high amounts of sugar at multiple meals per day is single-handedly driving diabetes, heart disease, lipid problems, strokes, cancer and other diseases across a large percentage of the populace. Of course a little here and there won't prove harmful or fatal, but consuming meal after meal of foods loaded with sugar can eventually lead to metabolic disease and obesity.

Sugar can hide behind many names on food labels, but it most often appears as "high fructose corn syrup." High fructose corn syrup is a cheap, processed sweetener that is commonly used to replace table sugar in processed foods. Food corporations even introduce sugar into baby formula, which may be hooking consumers to life-long sugar cravings.

Even natural sugars should be avoided or limited. If you think fruit juices, for example, are good for you, please reconsider. When you eat whole fruit you are ingesting supportive fiber, but when you drink fruit juice—even juice clearly labeled NO SUGAR ADDED—you get almost all sugar and little to no fiber. A grapefruit contains roughly three grams of fiber, but look at the nutrition info on a carton of grapefruit juice, and you'll see no fiber listed at all. You might as well drink a soda.

Indeed, juicing with fruit is not a good way to get lean. Without fiber to aid in digestion, your body releases insulin, the fat storage hormone.

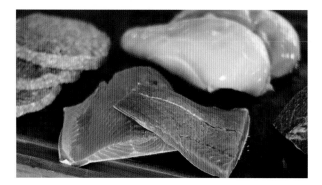

YOUR FOOD INTAKE

Food is fuel, and your food intake determines how we feel on the inside and how we look on the outside. But not all food is efficient fuel.

When devising a food intake plan that will transform their bodies, many people fail to consider the role of protein. Sure, the food pyramid and recommended daily allowances ascribe some semblance of space to this all-important macronutrient, but certainly not enough. Many "authorities" cite various carbohydrate and fat sources as mainstays of nutrition, but until you put protein at the forefront, you're not changing your body. Carbs and fats are just energy, calories that both allow and enable sustained movement. Protein, on the other hand, is what you are: it is flesh, and flesh is what you have control over to bring you your own complete physique. And please jettison the cry of "I don't want to get too big." It's simply not going to happen without the right combination of genetics, tons of weights hoisted on a consistent basis, an army of food and a lot of time.

YOUR CALORIC NEEDS

As I've previously stated, if you're eating mostly unprocessed foods, then you're generally going to stay lean. Having said that, and in the hopes of narrowing down just how much you should be consuming each day, here are some more specific guidelines for the three main nutritional macronutrients: protein, carbohydrates and fats.

Proteins

Consume 1 gram of protein per pound of body weight daily in the form of chicken and turkey breast, eggs, lean meats, fish or plant-based protein powders to maintain and build lean muscle mass. Protein, at 4 calories per gram, is composed of amino acids. To promote an anabolic, or muscle-building, state, you must consistently take in these building blocks of protein. Protein helps in the repair of tissues and in the ongoing process that results from muscle breakdown (from exercise) and muscle repair (from nutrition). A 200-pound man should take in roughly 200 grams of protein daily split among five small meals with approximately 40 grams per meal.

Carbohydrates

Consume roughly 1.5 grams of low-glycemic carbohydrates per pound of body weight on the days you work out in the form of beans, yams, quinoa,

THE GLYCEMIC INDEX

All carbohydrates are not equal to one another in terms of insulin release and fat storage. The Glycemic Index (GI) can help you track your carbohydrate intake, allowing you to gauge whether you are eating "good" or "bad" carbs. The GI tells you how quickly your blood-sugar levels rise after consuming certain kinds of carbohydrates. Look for carbohydrates with low GI scores ranking 55 or lower, and avoid those with high scores. White bread, white potatoes, white rice and alcoholic drinks have high GI score ratings of 70 or above. Medium-GI choices include muesli, oatmeal, and shredded wheat, rating 56 to 69. Low-GI foods include lentils, legumes, nuts and most vegetables, with scores of 55 or lower. Limit most dairy, soda, fruit juices, alcohol, breads and cereal, pasta, butter, margarine, heavy oils and fried food.

oatmeal, brown rice, whole- or sprouted-grain bread or legumes and roughly 1 gram on the days you do not. Carbs contain 4 calories per gram. You can consume fibrous carbs, such as salad greens and broccoli, in near limitless amounts due to their low caloric content.

Carbs can be classified into two main categories: simple and complex. Simple carbs are simple sugars that can be found in processed foods such as cakes, cookies and candy, as well as in more nutritious foods such as fruits and vegetables. Complex carbs are generally considered unrefined or unprocessed (during processing, nutrients are taken out to make for a longer shelf life). As previously discussed, ingesting mostly low-glycemic carbs is a major key to staying lean. A 200-pound man should take in roughly 250 grams of carbohydrates daily split among five small meals with approximately 50 grams per meal.

Fats

Consume roughly one-third of your body weight daily in the form of healthy oils like olive and coconut healthy fats found in such foods as nuts and avocados. Fats, at 9 calories per gram, are essential in the further acquisition of lean tissue and to regulate body functions. Skin and cell maintenance, eye and hair health, lowering of cholesterol levels and disease prevention are just some of the benefits of consuming the right kind of fats.

Fats can be further divided into subcategories including both saturated and unsaturated. The body doesn't digest saturated fats (bad fats) well and tends

to deposit them where they can build up, while unsaturated fats (good fats) are used for optimal health. A 200-pound man should take in roughly 65 grams of fat daily split among five small meals with approximately 13 grams per meal.

By totaling the grams from the three macronutrient groups you will arrive at your daily allotment of calories. It need not be exact and should not remain repeatedly the same foods—your intake should be changed now and then to offset boredom and further disarm the temptation to engage in emotional eating.

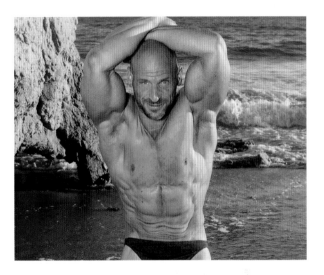

THE REAL KEY TO ABS

You might think that this section belongs in the chapter on exercise. After all, you've got to work your abs to make them show, right? As I say to new clients wanting to work just their abs and those convinced that the key to getting a trim and rippling midsection is crunches, sit-ups and more crunches, "Stop the crunches."

The key to tight abs is burning stored body fat through a reduced and quality nutritional intake and melting the fat off by elevating your metabolism through both weight training and cardio. Performing a set of squats rather than a set of crunches will do more to elevate your metabolism and the efficacy in which stored calories are utilized. I can prove it to you. Check your pulse after a set of squats and then check it after a set of crunches. It will be elevated after squats, especially if those squats were performed deep.

Want your abs to truly show? Stick to unprocessed foods, and consume them as soon after they are harvested as possible.

SUPPLEMENTATION

Supplements are, at best, supplemental to your intake. Filling nutritional gaps, helping to meet macronutrient levels, and offering ease and convenience are the major pluses of implementing sports supplementation. They should and will always take a backseat, however, to proper and complete whole foods.

In my competitive days and less hectic work life, I was able to get in my five regular meals with ease. Yet, like many, my adulthood added responsibilities that leave me with far less free time. The good news is that you can achieve outstanding results with limited time, either with or without supplements. I'm living proof: I got in shape for this book on an intake of three whole meals and two additional protein shakes daily.

Strangers, friends and even family often approach me with free samples of some new "miracle" supplement or stream of supplements. Then I am told how much extra income I can make by turning on my readers and clients to these products. Integrity is of utmost importance to me, and I have never hawked products to those who place continued trust in me simply to make a buck. Again, supplements will always be supplemental to food, and I only recommend something if I personally believe in it and take it. In truth we trust.

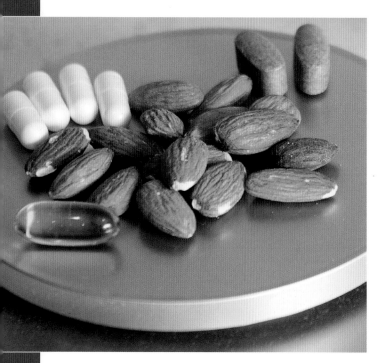

The list below, placed in order of each item's importance in my program, is exactly what I use in my arsenal, and I cite them for demonstration purposes only. As always with supplements, less is more, and more will never be better. I do not recommend supplements for everyone; these are merely what I take consistently to yield a quality physique to supplement my whole food intake and *Complete Physique* lifestyle.

Multivitamin packets

The multivitamin packet has always been my greatest insurance policy. Investing in your body through proper food intake and intense training must be supported by the underpinnings—in this case, vitamins and minerals. You could have the sturdiest steel beams, but without quality bolts, you'll never build a sound structure.

Many of us tend to consume the same or similar foods, and so multivitamins help to fill in the gaps. I take them every morning with breakfast.

Protein powders

Protein powders are an efficient way to fulfill your daily protein requirements. The greatest thing about protein powders is their portability, affordability and ability to supply a steady flow of this macronutrient to recovering muscles.

A casein-based powder is best taken at nighttime due to its slow digestion time, and whey-based powder is best consumed post-workout due to its immediate assimilation. These powders are also complete in all essential and nonessential amino acids, meaning that they have a high biological level, or BV (how well the body can both utilize and absorb a protein). I generally take protein powder with almonds (a good fat to slow down fast digestion) between whole-food meals.

Caffeine

Pretty much the first thing I reach for in the morning (following, of course, holding my dogs) is half a caffeine pill. Why not a cup of coffee or tea? I have nothing against the liquid stuff (provided it's not mixed with sugar and cream), but the pill just helps to get me going in the morning. Am I reliant on it? No. Is it an added boost to begin my morning? Absolutely. And I never take caffeine in any form after 4:00 p.m. to ensure adequate sleep.

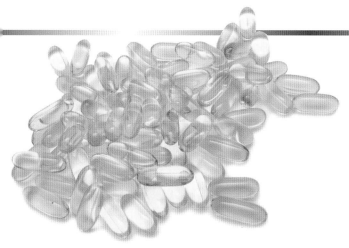

Fish oil

Fats and their many benefits are such an important weapon in the nutritional arsenal (when maintaining a low-fat intake) that they appear near the top of the list. Fish oil is a high-quality source of the healthy fats that help with metabolic and antioxidant support, smooth-functioning joint health and proper nervous system function. They are also great for the skin, hair and heart. They aid in dietary satiety and even help to improve your best lifts. I take one fish oil capsule at breakfast.

Pre-workout powders

Much like our smart phones today, pre-workout powders are everywhere. One wonders what we did to power our workouts before the invention of this ultra-popular category of supplements. Low in calories and meant to work in conjunction with whole foods, many pre-workout products contain caffeine for energy and focus, nitric oxide for an increased muscle pump, creatine for fuller muscles and increased endurance, and other stimulants. These products are strong, so if you are sensitive to stimulants and/or have high blood pressure, stay clear of them. It is also a good idea to only take a pre-workout powder for limited periods or cycle different kinds to counteract their diminishing effects over time. I alternate brands weekly. I take it minutes before my workout with a meal.

Glucosamine/chondroitin

Depending on to whom you speak, this supplement either works wonders or does nothing. I take it at least for the mental boost, knowing that my joints are strong and connective tissues and cartilage supported. It gives me the mental confidence to perform my best in the gym during the rigors of heavy lifting. When I don't take this supplement for a few days, I can definitely feel a difference. Joints are subject to heavy loads and repetitive motion during lifting, and this product supports the production of synovial fluid within the bone tissue. I take two with my first meal.

Branched-chain amino acids (BCAA)

Out of 22 amino acids, the building blocks of protein, 9 are essential and must be derived from food because your body cannot produce them. BCAAs contain the three most important of the amino acids: leucine, isoleucine and valine, which are responsible for protein synthesis (the process whereby individual muscle cells increase in size), energy production and to prevent or decrease muscle breakdown. I take four capsules prior to breakfast in conjunction with caffeine every morning in order to keep a muscle-preserving and even anabolic, or growing, state, especially when I'm on a restricted caloric intake.

THE ROLE OF HORMONES

The release of varying hormones plays a large role in determining the body's muscular composition. Testosterone increases muscle protein synthesis, the process by which our muscles grow. It is released from the testicles in males and to a lesser degree from the ovaries in females. Growth hormone is what allows us to grow from children into adults and helps to keep us youthful as well as stimulate muscle tissue repair. It is secreted from the pituitary gland. Insulin, as discussed earlier, helps to assist nourishment into muscle cells. It is produced in the pancreas. These three powerful hormones are anabolic in nature, that is, muscle building.

The equally powerful but derailing hormone cortisol is opposite in effect in that it is catabolic, meaning it breaks down muscle tissue. Cortisol is released by the adrenal glands in times of both mental and physical stress as a coping mechanism. Too much can lead to gaining fat and losing muscle, the exact opposite of our intentions here.

It is nearly impossible to halt or block cortisol release, but it is possible to lessen its effects on your body by including regular exercise in your lifestyle. Endorphins trigger positive feelings within the body and are released from both resistance training and aerobic exercise and will help to lower your cortisol levels. Deep sleep is unique in that this is when your cortisol levels are at their lowest and your growth hormone is at its highest.

THE PORTABLE KITCHEN

Time and time again when I inquire about my clients' nutrition during work hours, I hear the reply, "I have no time to pack food to take with me, and all that's available is x, y and z." Of course, x, y and z are always poor choices. Without trying to lecture them like a parent scolding a child, I remind everyone that we all lead busy lives, and, truly, as the saying goes, "Failing to prepare is preparing to fail."

It really doesn't take that much time to fire up the grill or saucepan and cook chicken while scooping protein powder into shaker cups and portioning frozen rice and veggies into storage containers for transport to the office. Let's assume that these days most of us have a microwave at work, and so . . . there you go.

I may be a trainer who spends many hours in the gym five days per week helping my clients to achieve their physique goals, but believe me when I tell you that between scheduling them, I do get in both my workouts and clean meals, and so too should you make healthy eating one of your priorities. And no matter your vocational situation, you can make this happen. Going to work without prepared food is like going into battle with guns but no bullets.

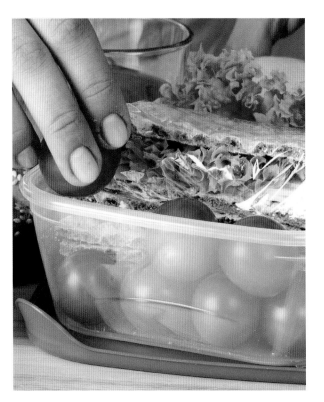

EATING OUT

Whether it be business, travel or a date, most of us are eating out often and are more likely to consume more calories than when we eat at home. And those calories are likely to come from heavy starches such as rice, breads and pastas, as opposed to vegetables and leafy greens. As I've said before, there's almost nowhere that you can't find a healthier alternative when in public. Of course, most of us have been in a situation where someone reminds us to live a little and to put the tuna and carrots down and dig in. And from time to time, we should.

I've certainly been on my share of dates, meetings, parties and other events at which I couldn't dig in—I had competition plans or a scheduled photo shoot that prevented me from indulging, but even this was only for a limited time. When those plans concluded, it was back to indulging here and there, all the while keeping myself within striking distance of a complete physique. Not giving in to peer pressure is one thing, but not living is another matter entirely.

The *Complete Physique* plan gives you a bag of tools that will help you to maintain a livable, long-term lifestyle that is above all else, attainable. The goal on paper is to become your best. But the real-world goal is to get there while navigating this thing called life, while anticipating problems and offering solutions, before they occur. And for any fitness plan, eating out is a problem with many solutions.

Mexican restaurant

You may think of Mexican as just fried tortillas, heavy cheeses and frozen margaritas, but when eating Mexican, you can't go wrong with white chicken fajitas, black beans or pinto beans, soft whole-wheat tortillas, salsa and a negligible amount of guacamole. Watch the calorie-dense sour cream, cheeses, chips and tortillas.

Sushi restaurant

Sushi restaurants offer lots of healthy selections. If available, ask for brown rice rolls, and avoid deep-fried tempura dishes. Stick to less fancy, less dressed, cleaner rolls such as salmon, tuna, shrimp, yellowtail or veggie rolls. Watch out for hidden ingredients, such as mayonnaise, which can be found in spicy tuna rolls. To feel more satiated, start with either the miso soup, edamame or a mixed green salad devoid of heavy dressing.

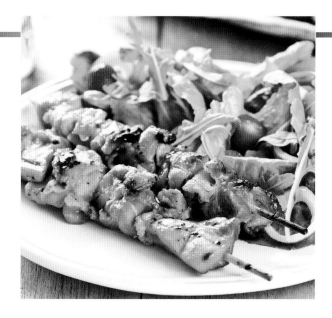

Mediterranean restaurant

A Mediterranean restaurant is another venue that offers lots of healthy choices. Order chicken kabobs or chicken without the skin with various grilled vegetables. Olive oil is the main source of fat used in this cuisine, which consists of largely unprocessed foods, but steer clear of the fried falafel and pita bread. Go for moderate hummus and moderate rice. Watch the fat-laden spreads and dips. Enjoy spiced onions, tomatoes and pickles.

Thai restaurant

Rich Thai curries are delicious, but loaded with calories and saturated fat. Order a dish that is steamed and is devoid of coconut milk. Cashew chicken is a good choice, because cashews contain plenty of healthy fats, and the dish can be complemented with brown rice. Hot and sour soup is another low-calorie, low-fat option, but keep in mind that it's high in sodium. As a starter, choose steamed spring rolls filled with healthy vegetables.

Indian restaurant

Indian restaurants offer numerous options for a clean intake. It's a flavorful cuisine, containing many spices, some of which have been shown to contain beneficial antioxidants. Lean foods such as Tandoori chicken or shrimp are good choices. Skip the high-glycemic naan, the deep-fried poori and the griddle-fried paratha breads, and opt for the whole-wheat roti. Vegetarians can also eat clean by having legume-based dishes, but just avoid the heavy sauces.

Coffee shop

These days it is hard to avoid the ubiquitous coffee shops that have popped up on nearly every street corner. If you find yourself in one, ignore the high-calorie frappuccinos and flavored lattes, which are loaded with fat and sugar, and opt for plain tea or coffee. These shops used to sell just coffee, but now offer a host of breakfast and lunch items, too. Go for a whole-grain oatmeal (and stir in your favorite protein powder) or a reduced-fat turkey sandwich on a whole-wheat English muffin (tell them to hold the cheese).

Buffet

Let's face it, when on the *Complete Physique* plan, a buffet restaurant is probably not the place to be—mounds of all-you-can eat selections are just invitations to gluttony. Still, even at a buffet you can gather a plate of salad, vegetables and fruit. Assume lean protein (other than hard-boiled eggs) is nonexistent at these places, but count on fried chicken. Simply grab a breast, and discard the skin and fried parts. You will then have a supreme source of first-class lean protein.

Deli

Skip the mile-high layers of pastrami or corned beef, and go for a lean meat such as turkey, chicken or roast beef on whole-wheat bread with vegetables and a low-calorie condiment such as mustard.

Convenience stores

Most of the "quickie-mart" road stops are stocked with RTDs (ready-to-drink meal replacements). In addition, there is beef or turkey jerky, which is very low in fat, despite its high sodium content. Various trail mixes and single pieces of fruit are also good choices. Remember that you can find a way to eat clean, even while fueling up at the gas pump.

Vegetarian restaurant

Vegetarian restaurants offer a host of clean choices. For one, there's soybeans, which by themselves contain all the essential amino acids (building blocks of protein), and for another, there's quinoa, a near-perfect food. There's also legumes, nuts and grains. Keep in mind that the label VEGETARIAN by itself does not mean "healthy" or "lean," because even veggie dishes can be prepared by frying. Opt for grilled dishes without heavy sauces or condiments.

THE VEGETARIAN'S PLAN

Although vegetarianism has been around for millennia, it was not until the nineteenth and twentieth centuries that it truly grew in the Western world. In our century, vegetarianism in its many forms, from raw veganism, which includes only fresh and uncooked fruit, nuts, seeds and vegetables, to ovo-lacto vegetarianism, which includes animal/dairy products such as eggs, milk and honey, continues to grow and flourish.

Along with paying close attention to what they eat, vegetarians of all stripes are just as conscious about getting into peak shape (if not more so) as their carnivorous counterparts are. Whatever your food preferences and lifestyle, the *Complete Physique* plan is for you. You can hone your body to its absolute best, with maximal lean muscle and minimal body fat, consuming a diet of only foods grown from the earth and none that originate with a face.

One of the biggest misconceptions about an exclusively plant-based intake is that it does not supply your body with enough protein, or complete protein sources. Yet, most plant foods do contain protein to some measure. Take, for example, spinach: Its protein per calorie equals that of chicken, though there are indeed far fewer calories per ounce in spinach than there are in chicken. You would have to eat a lot more spinach to get an equivalent amount of protein.

Plant proteins are just as valuable as those found in animal sources. The main difference is that animal sources are whole, meaning that they contain all the essential amino acids, the building blocks of protein. You can, however, still build an amazing physique on a plant-based intake, as long as you carefully combine foods to get all the essential amino acids.

If you are consuming a rich variety of plant-based foods—seeds such as quinoa (naturally high in protein), fruits, legumes, nuts and leafy green vegetables—and in ample amounts, you will likely take in enough complete sources of protein. You also derive other benefits. The natural fiber found in these unprocessed, whole foods (unlike their meat counterparts) aid in digestion, and they actually help to keep you lean because many of these foods are nutrient dense, low in calories and full of vitamins and antioxidants. They also tend to be cheaper and less perishable than meat.

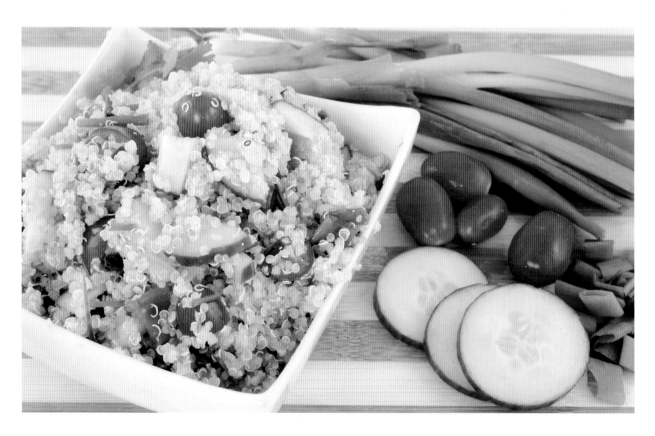

SAMPLE DAY/VEGETARIAN

The following sample training day's clean intake provides roughly the type and quantity of nutrients a vegetarian needs. Feel free to change the times and even sequence of the meals if it better suits you.

MEAL 1
8:00 a.m.
- plant protein powder
- oats
- unsweetened almond milk
- berries

MEAL 2
11:00 a.m.
- bowl of quinoa
- kale and raw nuts
- green salad with vegetables

MEAL 3
2:00 p.m.
(pre-workout meal)
- smoothie done in water with soy protein powder, raw greens and fruit

MEAL 4
5:00 p.m.
(post-workout meal)
- brown rice
- half an avocado
- beans
- green salad with vegetables

MEAL 5
8:00 p.m.
- legumes with kale
- butternut squash
- green vegetables

On the flip side, many of the benefits of plant-based foods come with an added expense of high carbs, most especially the sugars found in fruit. Limit these type of carbs in order to get lean and also to prevent such diseases as type 2 diabetes. Having said that, if you're eating plant-based, the chances are still high that you will get enough of everything you need, and virtually none of what you do not. You may even require fewer nutritional supplements.

The general consensus is that we don't need as much protein as we were once told, but to build or even maintain muscle mass, you're going to need an adequate protein intake on a daily basis—roughly a gram (at least) of protein per pound of lean body weight every day. That means a 200-pound man who carries 180 lean pounds of muscle needs a minimum of 180 grams of protein per day to maintain muscle mass—and even more is he wants to build new tissue. A plant-based intake is generally low in calories, but taking in enough calories to get sufficient protein is key, provided the foods are low glycemic, so as to minimize and negate the release of insulin, the fat storage hormone. For this reason, including plant-based protein powders like rice or soy in your diet is a good idea to help supplement your intake and hit your daily numbers.

MORE THAN JUST TOFU & SALADS

There's so much more to a vegetarian diet than the stereotypically limited tofu and salads. Indeed, plant-based nutrition can be delicious, different and varied.

If you follow a plant-based diet, be sure to choose from all of its four main food groups: whole grains, beans, vegetables and fruits. Low-glycemic starches include healthy pastas, brown rice, vegan wraps and tortillas and oats. Many vegetables, including portobello mushrooms, kale, spinach, romaine lettuce and sweet potatoes, are nutrient-dense and vitamin-fortified foods that will help to keep you lean. Additionally, gluten-free options can greatly help those with allergies and those suffering from celiac disease.

The time factor in preparing plant-based meals can be of further benefit,—it takes mere minutes to put together a dish such as quinoa, mushrooms, spinach, tomatoes, broccoli and a handful of raw nuts. Another meal could be a veggie burger in vegan bread, such as Ezekiel, with leafy greens and golden beets. A protein-and-vitamin-rich smoothie takes mere seconds. When on the go, pack raw nuts, fruits, vegetables and grains in baggies or storage containers to keep you on track and progressing.

Consuming an array of unprocessed plant-based foods throughout the day portioned into small meals that are loaded with fiber will help you get lean and stay healthy. Limit packaged foods that have labels listing a surplus of unpronounceable ingredients, and be sure to take advantage of low-calorie spices and low-glycemic condiments to add extra flavor to an already colorful plate.

THE CHEAT MEAL

What is the cheat meal, and why should you add it to your food intake plan? It is simply one extravagant meal that you indulge in once a week, which will actually reset both your metabolism and state of mind.

Don't force one if you don't think it's warranted, but if you go for it, don't let a cheat meal morph into a cheat day, as it often does. It doesn't mean gorging over the weekend only to reset on Monday. It's really *just one meal a week* in which to elevate your calories and enjoy the foods you've been limiting or even avoiding. If you can have it early in the day, great. This gives you a chance to use up some of that ingested energy.

For some, the cheat meal is a social thing. Maybe that upcoming wedding is your indulgent reward to yourself. For others (like myself), it's often a private thing to be enjoyed in the sanctity of home. It's up to you—choose the time and place and lose yourself for that one meal. And then get back on track, guilt-free.

THE FINAL 10

My hope for you is that you use the knowledge within this book to achieve your personal best. When you're getting close—meaning your clothes are fitting well and there's some abdominal definition going on—the final 10 pounds can prove quite an annoyance. Your instinct might be to do more activity and take in less food, but extreme measures do not always guarantee success. And they often backfire.

Sometimes all you need to do is to take a closer look at your current behaviors. Are you taking in hidden sugars? I know you're eating skinless chicken breasts, but are you using excessive ketchup or other sugar-laden condiments to get them down? Are you eating ground turkey or ground turkey breast? The turkey breast is far leaner. Greek yogurt is a complete and fantastic source of protein, but how much sugar is listed on the label? Are you using butter to prepare your eggs? Are you having a glass of wine just about every night? The cream and sweetener, no matter how slight, in your morning coffee adds up over time.

But let's assume that it's all clean eating. Sometimes it's simply a matter of time. So go easy on yourself. You're probably doing enough, so just keep doing it, and be patient. You didn't get out of shape in a matter of days and you won't get back into shape in the same time frame. Just keep on the road to results. You'll be showing a beach-worthy body at the end of the journey.

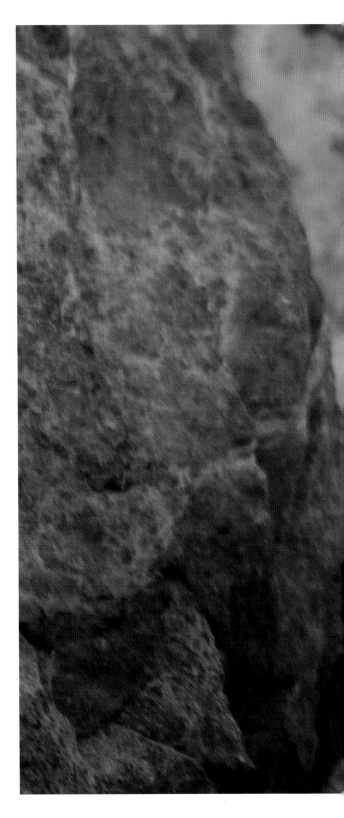

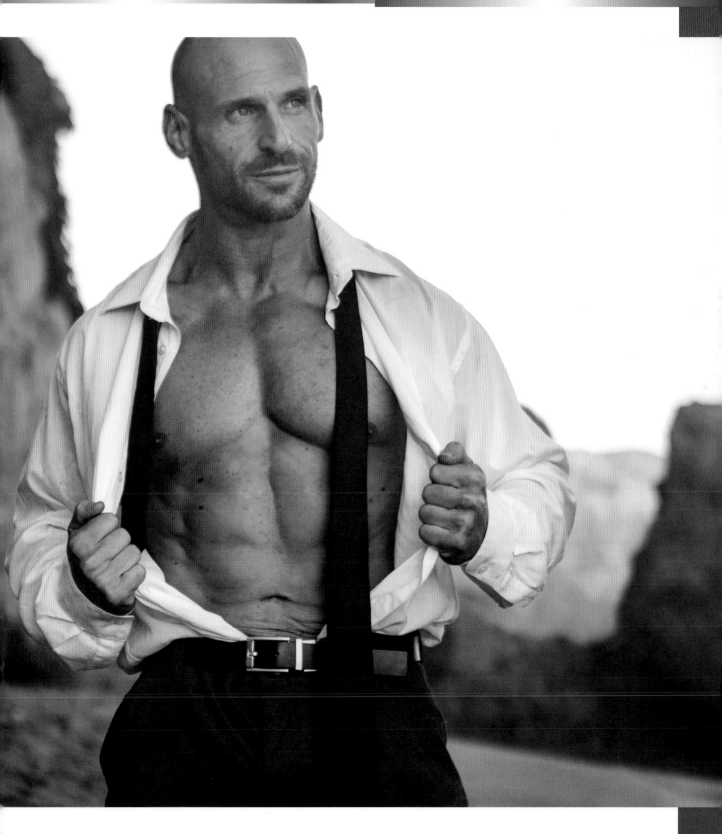

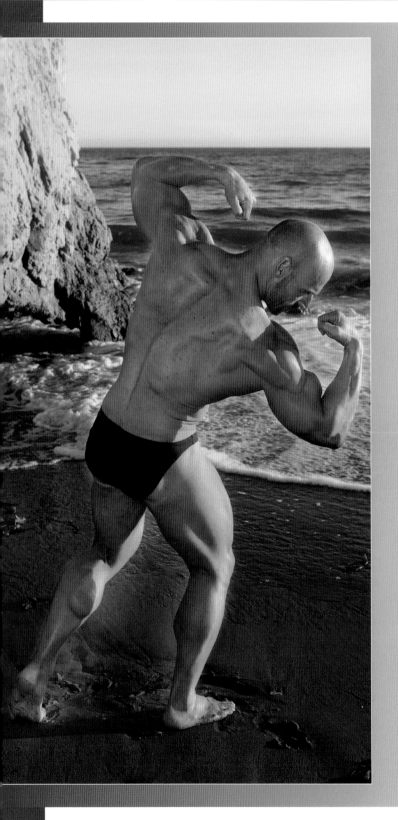

PREPARING FOR THE BIG DAY: PEAKING SECRETS FOR THE FINAL WEEK OF YOUR JOURNEY

The great thing about your transformation is that it is a solo endeavor, a private journey in which you are bettering your previous best, and no one else's. We are all different, with differing fitness levels, yet with the common goal of besting ourselves, so our targeted question is not "Will you get to the top of the mountain?" but "When?"

As a trainer told me long ago, if you're not ready one week out from an event, all the little tweaking and adjusting in the world won't do much to change your physique. There are, however, "peaking secrets" that I've used with success over the years, and they have made a difference to my appearance. Many of you are using the *Complete Physique* plan to actually get in shape for an event on a specific date—a wedding, reunion, beach vacation—so I am laying down exactly what I did in the last week to prepare for my big event.

My event, the photo shoot for this book, was to take place over a weekend, with Saturday being specified as my main peaking day, so I began final preparation on the prior Monday. From Monday through Wednesday I willingly and voluntarily salted my foods (which I wouldn't recommend if you are prone to high blood pressure). The theory behind this is that the extra salt will retain water in the skin, giving it a smooth, almost bloated look . . . temporarily.

On Tuesday, I had a full-body wax to provide ample time for my skin to heal and for any swelling to go down. I also practiced isometrics or muscle posing for five minutes per day all seven days of this last week. Nothing fancy, just traditional bodybuilding poses you'd see in nearly any muscle magazine. That gave me greater control over the muscles of my body, allowing me to tense these muscles while still relaxing my facial muscles. This way, my physique would appear super hard, but my expressions wouldn't be tense or forced.

My workouts were the same as those prescribed during Phase 3 of the *Complete Physique* plan with an extra day of cardio thrown in early Saturday morning. I did this more for a mental boost rather than any physical change for the big day.

Come Thursday, I then cut out as much sodium as possible, eating my foods with no condiments or seasonings. I also added in asparagus (a natural diuretic) all the while drinking a lot of water in an effort to flush the salt from my body and make my skin appear tighter.

Friday was a full-body spray tan. And then, Saturday, I woke up fresh and ready to go, although I still drank plenty of water to stay hydrated. We began shooting outdoors under the sun, which caused even more subcutaneous water loss—so much so that by the time we were ready to snap the interior shots, my physique was at its absolute peak.

Worth mentioning is the fact that I had carbs even with my last meal. Many people opt to cut their carbs after an afternoon meal, but this is simply too drastic and unrealistic. You need those carbs to perform demanding resistance training and cardiovascular exercise week in and week out while attempting to hold onto precious muscle tissue and jettison stored body fat. If you attempt to cut carbs too early in your day, you will most assuredly binge later on or late at night. Remember, if you follow a diet you will ultimately and permanently fail. If you live a lifestyle you will consistently succeed.

You will lose fat and gain lean muscle during your program, so be wary of the scale; it does not give a true indication of what's really going on behind the number and underneath the threads. Although experience and results dictate that I am not a proponent of numbers—that is, I am not concerned with sheer body weight but rather the composition of that body weight and how it looks—I did, however, weigh myself when I began the *Complete Physique* plan and then again on the day of the photo shoot. I began at 242 pounds and ended at 198 pounds. My goal this time was twofold: to come in with a little more lean muscle and even less body fat than my previous books.

Aside from increasing my lifts on target sets, I upped my protein a little from the previous plan and allotted myself one cheat meal per week until six weeks out from the photo shoot. I then eliminated all cheat meals until after the shoot. Then I slipped back into a maintenance mode. My suggestions are to use your clothes, the mirror and your pictures to assess your true condition.

SAMPLE PEAKING MENU

Here is a sample of a daily menu (with supplementation included) that I followed as I prepared for the photos for this book.

MORNING SUPPLEMENTATION
7:00 a.m.
- 4 BCAA (branched chain amino acids) pills
- 1/2 caffeine pill

MEAL 1
8:00 a.m.
- 1 multivitamin/mineral pack
- 1 fish oil tablet
- 2 chondroitin/glucosamine tablets
- 2 whole eggs and 8 egg whites, scrambled and topped with salsa or hot sauce
- 1 cup ready-made oatmeal with one Splenda and ground cinnamon

MEAL 2
11:00 a.m.
- 1 scoop pre-workout powder
- 2 scoops of casein protein powder in water with half an avocado

MEAL 3
2:00 p.m.
- 2 grilled chicken breasts seasoned with garlic powder
- 1 yam
- asparagus

MEAL 4
5:00 p.m.
- 2 scoops of casein/whey protein powder and a small handful of raw almonds blended in water

MEAL 5
8:00 p.m.
- 2 tilapia fillets seasoned with Cajun spice
- ready-made brown rice bowl with a few drops of Worcestershire sauce
- asparagus

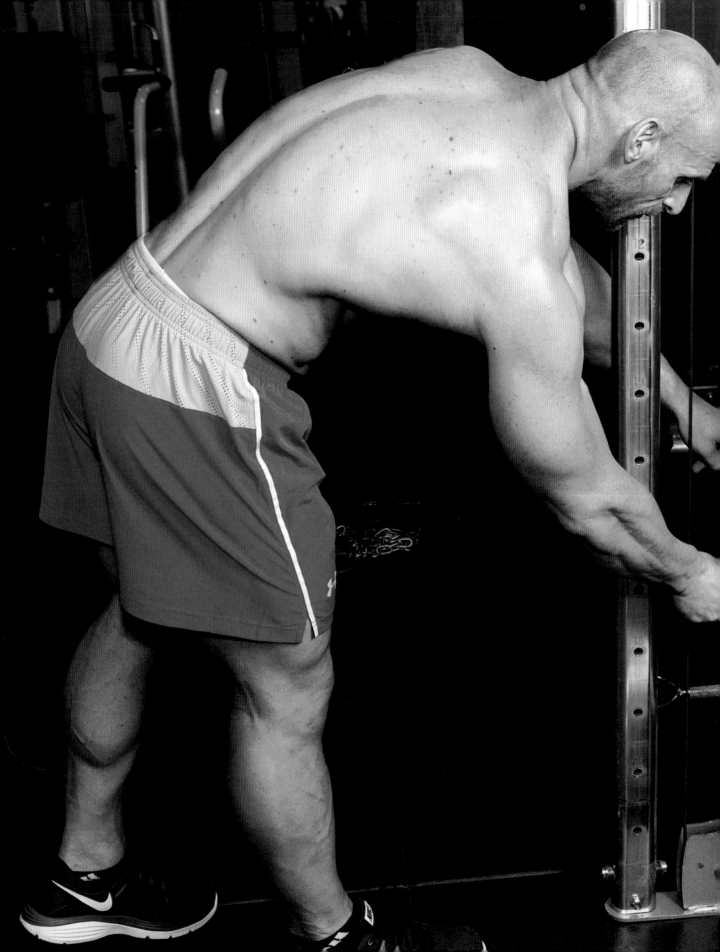

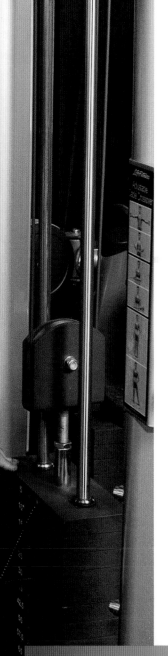

5 NUTS, BOLTS & BARBELLS

My personal training clients often ask me why I choose a certain exercise or why I couple or group things the way I do. It has never made sense to me to hear someone say, "It's this way because I say it is." If I can't supply the reason why, then it's not of much benefit. So, here I answer many of the questions I'm often asked. I've also included the phrases that I often recite to my clients to help them properly fire from the target muscles—let's call them "Hollisisms."

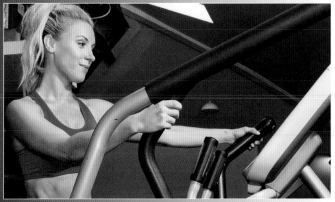
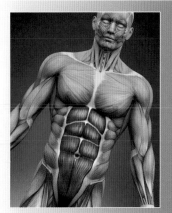
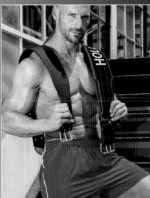

THE WHAT

You will see in the following pages that describe the exercises and how to do them that I've grouped the exercises according to their target muscles. Just what are these major muscles' true functions—not just when we work out, but as we move through everyday life, as well? And what are the key exercises that will target these muscles or groups of them?

Chest: *pectoralis major*
Function: This thick, fan-shaped muscle of the chest draws the arm across the front of the body.
Key exercise: Incline Dumbbell Flye
Hollisism: "Crush an imaginary finger between your chest to feel your chest muscles contract."

Back: *latissimus dorsi*
Function: This broad muscle of the back pulls the arm downward towards the pelvis and also stabilizes the torso during movement.
Key exercise: Neutral-Grip Pulldown
Hollisism: "Elbow behind you to feel the lats contract."

Shoulders: *deltoids*
Function: These muscles form the rounded contour of the shoulder and facilitate the 360-degree rotation of the arm away from the body.
Key exercise: Smith Machine Shoulder Press
Hollisism: "Down slow, up aggressive."

Biceps: *biceps brachii*
Function: A two-headed muscle that lies on the upper arm works to shorten the arm towards the shoulder (flexion) and turns the hand from palms down to palms up (supination).
Key exercise: Reverse Barbell Curl
Hollisism: "Keep your elbows in, and curl the farthest arc away from you."

Triceps: *triceps brachii*
Function: This three-headed muscle at the back of the upper arm extends the elbow (extension) and turns the hand from palms up to palms down (pronation).
Key exercise: Reverse-Grip Pushdown
Hollisism: "Keep your elbows in, and come up no higher than 90 degrees."

Quadriceps: *vastus medialis, vastus intermedius, vastus lateralis, rectus femoris*
Function: This large group of muscles at the front of the thigh extends or straightens the knee.
Key exercise: Front Squat
Hollisism: "Push through your heels down into hell to get yourself back up."

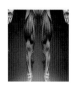

Hamstrings: *biceps femoris, semitendinosus and semimembranosus*
Function: This group of muscles at the back of the thigh brings the heel toward the buttocks (knee flexion).
Key exercise: One-legged Swiss Ball Leg Curl
Hollisism: "Pelvis up, dig your heels into the ball like a claw and draw it in strong."

Calves: *gastrocnemius*
Function: This powerful bipennate muscle lies on the back of the calf and elevates the heels.
Key exercise: Seated Calf Raise
Hollisism: "Toes straight on, down slow, up aggressive."

Abdominals: *rectus abdominis*
Function: This group of stomach muscles flexes the spine by bringing the rib cage toward the pelvis.
Key exercise: Twisting Crunch
Hollisism: "Pull from the belly button, not the neck."

THE WHY

For you to claim your own complete physique, you must have a plan. The *Complete Physique* plan calls for a three-phase program of only four hours of resistance training per week. Why does it work? Wouldn't it be better to work everything twice a week? Wouldn't it be more effective to work biceps before a larger group like chest? Why can't I just do cardio first and then do my weight training?

Over time, and with consistency, you will be able to generate a higher level of intensity than was previously possible. This is a principle that works for both the mental and physical. Math equations become easier the more experience you have with them. A tree will fall with fewer skilled swings from an axe wielded by a lumberjack than it will from the haphazard chops of the neophyte who just picked up an axe at the nearest hardware store.

You must be absolutely present during your workouts—meaning that you are focused on what you are doing and giving your workout your complete attention. You must concentrate on hitting the correct muscles for the exercise and stay intent on progressing. If you do these things, then the four hours of actual resistance training will always be enough work.

The workouts in this book are tough, and if you're able to train each muscle group twice per week, rather than the once the program calls for, then two things become immediately apparent: if you still have more in tank, you didn't train hard enough, and you're at risk of overtraining. Training before you are fully recovered from your previous workout will leave you tired and weak with flat-looking muscles. Overtraining also saps motivation, which can set you back, and even might result in injury. Once per week is plenty—just make each session count.

As to why I've set the workouts in the order they appear—sure, you could conceivably work biceps before chest. It isn't necessarily wrong, but when training two or more muscle groups in one session, it's best to start with the larger muscle because it will generally use the smaller muscle as an ancillary, or helper, muscle during execution. This warms up the smaller for the more direct work to follow. If you trained your biceps before your chest then your biceps would be so engorged with blood—or the pump as bodybuilders call it—that your range of motion might be compromised due to an inflexibility within your upper arms. When it comes to progressive change, we need a full and complete range of motion during each and every exercise.

The question, "Why do you list cardio after weight training—doesn't it usually come before?" is a common one. If you perform cardio before your weights, you will essentially be too tired for the resistance portion of the program. Weight training is reliant on glycogen, or stored carbohydrates, for energy, and cardio is fueled by adipose, or stored fat. Two different fuels for two different activities. Don't believe it? Try one workout doing weights and then cardio, and then the next week reverse that order for the same day of muscle groupings. Tell me which day was more productive.

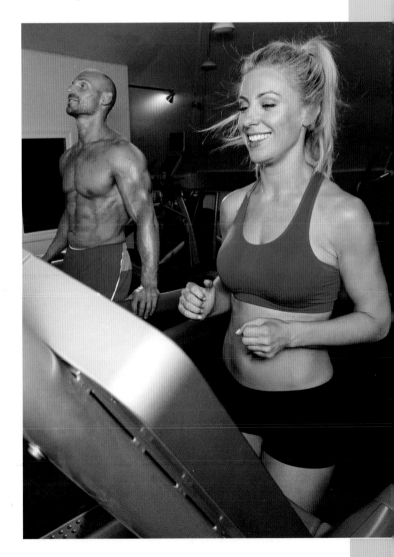

THE ANGLE OF SUCCESS

In both my mind and practice, training for aesthetics (how a muscle looks) as opposed to functionality (how a muscle performs) is largely about the angles. Take the game of pool for example. Success is based on angles. What angle will allow you to get the ball in

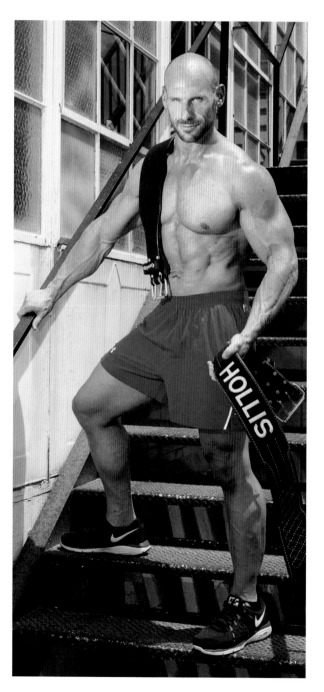

from a particular shot? The same can be said for your endeavors here. What angles will it take to develop the muscle from all sides and make it complete? This is why learning how to get in peak shape from a former bodybuilder, someone who was and is foremost concerned with developing the body for its own sake and not solely in terms of how strongly it can perform, is vital to your success. We are concerned here not with making you appear skinny in clothing but in truly being lean out of it.

If your foremost concern is performance, then our approach would be somewhat different. But when was the last time you attended a reunion and someone asked how far you could hit the ball? If you're like me, then you'd rather hear how amazing you're looking.

MIND-TO-MUSCLE CONNECTION

Often talked about, but not really explained, the mind-to-muscle connection is that ability to connect with the weights from the very first set and actually feel the correct muscles firing.

For example, compare a gym-goer concerned with working the chest who pumps out rep after perfect rep under the bar during the bench press, whose chest seems to rise with each completed repetition, with another gym-goer—this one arches the back and pushes more with the shoulders and arms and far less than with the actual muscle in the spotlight—the chest—just to cross it off the list and say it was done. The mind-to-muscle connection is so powerful that it separates two gym types: the person with the actual development in his or her chest, and the other person with a flat, almost concave, chest and overdeveloped front shoulders and triceps.

Fear not if this sounds new or unusual to you, for this ability is learned over time. Now that you know what your muscles do, you have a head start in properly using them during your exercises. When I began working out at age 13, it took me two years to feel my chest working and even longer to properly isolate my back—and they eventually became two of my strongest and most developed body parts. They helped me win a national title at 19.

The mind-to-muscle connection cannot be rushed: it must be primed. If you race through your workouts, you will quickly exhaust your reserves and miss out from garnering the best results. Think of downing a hot coffee. It gets down, but you're not really tasting it, and you risk burning your throat.

LIFE AT THE GYM

Although the *Complete Physique* plan is, at its core, self-building, you're going to do most of that building at the gym or fitness center. During my lifetime, I've spent more hours in gyms either training myself or helping others than I've spent in classrooms—and that is a serious amount of time. I've learned what to wear, how to navigate the rules, how to prevent accidents or injury and how to peacefully and happily coexist with my fellow gym-goers.

Gym etiquette—it's really just a matter of using your common sense and common courtesy.

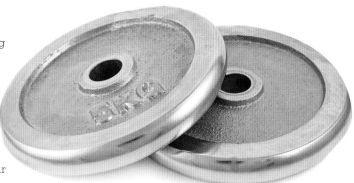

Attire

When it comes to gym clothing and support, try to wear what is, above all else, comfortable. And if it looks good too, well, then that's just an added bonus. But the gym is no place to stage a fashion show. You are *in* the gym so that you look good *out* of it.

When I work out, I like to see what muscles I am working, without being too showy. If it's leg day then I'm in shorts. If it's upper body, a V-neck T-shirt does the job nicely. Layering to sweat out excess water is not a good idea—the water will only be replaced later, and you are in the gym to lose body fat, not weight and certainly not water weight.

Ultra-restrictive compression wear makes a bold statement, but if you're not in tip-top shape, every flaw will be on glaring display. For some, this is actually motivating, but I save the compression wear for when I am in top shape.

Wear sneakers that have support, especially those with gel. A shoe with no support or nearly flat-heeled is going to make a leg day workout feel even tougher than it already is.

Respect

It doesn't matter how far along you are or how developed your physique, be kind and respectful to others in the gym. A sense of entitlement or superiority doesn't belong in our world, and by "our world," I refer to the domain in which we better ourselves: the gym, our safe place. Whether you're event ready and hitting posing shots with your shirt off in the middle of the room, or overweight and underconfidant as you set foot inside for the first time, the gym is the great equalizer. It doesn't matter if you're a millionaire or facing hard times, in the gym you get out what you put out. My advice: Be cool to everybody.

Re-rack weights

If you're strong enough to lift it, then you're strong enough to rack it. No one needs to navigate through a minefield of iron in order to get his or her next set in or to pull dozens of 45-pound plates off the leg press machine. Don't feel like racking? No problem. Just stick to the machines.

Always use protection

Whether squatting or bench pressing, it takes seconds to fasten the collars on the bar, and even less time for an accident to occur when the plates slide off. There's nothing masculine or cool or herculean about lifting without protection. Buckle up.

Let others work in

Oftentimes someone is using what I consider key pieces of equipment: the incline press, the Smith machine or leg press, and I'll kindly inquire how many sets are left. If the answer is "Just one or two," I'll wait it out. But then there is the answer that boils my blood a little: "I don't know yet." I wait a bit to see if that persons invites me to work in with him or her—as this is the appropriate response—but rarely do I hear it from the "I don't knowers." So I pay it forward, always inviting someone to work in when asked how many sets I have left. My advice: Don't hog the equipment.

Be mindful of space

I work out of a trainer's gym where peripheral vision and knowledge of space is important in order to avoid injury and to exercise just plain old-professional courtesy. Numerous times I've nearly been kicked in the face by gym-goers swinging their legs back and forth and up and down. Remember—it's not a private backyard, it's a group gym.

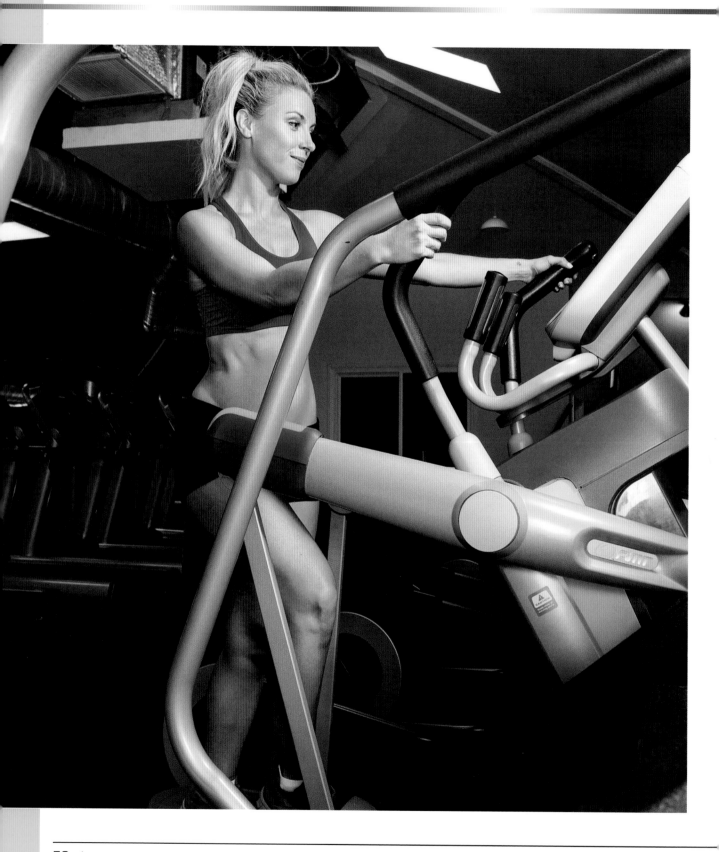

Ask for a spot

Many times I've looked over to see someone pinned under a barbell and left trying to roll it off his or her chest. After I rescue the person, I give my advice: never hesitate to ask for a spot. It's not worth an accident. Someone is always available. Just don't put on so much weight that the spotter is doing most of the work.

Never interrupt a set

Whether you're lifting 10 pounds or 100 pounds, once a set begins, finish it, and let others do the same. When I'm working with a client or training myself, finishing a set is like a surgeon in progress. You wouldn't interrupt a surgeon, and the same should be said about anyone working out. As the surgeon betters his patient through skillful maneuvering, we better ourselves in the gym through skillful lifting.

Don't be (overtly) naked

In every gym that I've ever been in, there's always that one guy who is not only comfortable naked, but also displaying his nakedness while conversing with others. Of course showering in the gym is perfectly normal, but people's feelings about nudity vary wildly. Me? I don't really need to see some guy's underpinnings while chatting about last night's game.

Of all the cardio machines . . .

With rows and rows of vacant cardio machines, why does that person have to choose the one right next to yours? Sure it's his or her right, but why set up shop right next to you with loud phone conversations, heavy breathing, rattling keys, and, oh yes, drinks? My advice: Unless the gym is packed, pick a machine that puts some space between you and the other gym-goer.

Don't leave valuables lying around

Unfortunately, locker break-ins are a regular occurrence in nearly every gym I've ever been in. It may look silly, but I always keep my keys, wallet and iPad (for reading during cardio), on my person at all times when in a gym—any gym.

Don't touch your face

Never touch your face in a gym. Too many gym-goers do not wash their hands after using the restroom and then proceed to touch the equipment. This message has been brought to you by the letters S, A, F, and E . . . you're welcome.

Moaning and screaming

Labored breathing, a tad extra vocal *oomph* on a last rep or two, sure, but those gym-goers who seem to moan and scream, whether consciously or unconsciously drawing attention to themselves, are both distracting and unnecessary. The loudest person in the room is the weakest person in the room, both physically and, more important, mentally. Save the sound effects for the bedroom.

Don't stare

Maybe it's okay at a boxing match, in a classroom or at the parade, but staring in the gym is a no-no. Either to the same or opposite sex, it's just rude. The only thing you should stare at in the gym is into space or in a mirror, because you need your focus and a clear head to advance toward a productive next set. Besides, other gym-goers notice when you're focused, and this too can often go over well.

Gas

Indeed, sometimes nature does run its course as evidenced during the descent of a squat, leg press or crunch, but forcing it out while others breathe the musty air is a definite no-no. Lest you think you can get away with it on the lone treadmill or stairmaster, someone will usually walk right into it like a deer in headlights—and that person will know it was you.

Wipe down benches machines

It's tough enough to find a vacated bench in modern-day gyms, and the last thing you need is to lie in someone else's sweat angels. Even if you have to use your own shirt (provided it's not sweaty), please wipe down benches and machine after use.

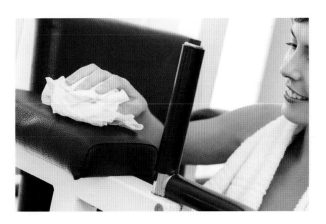

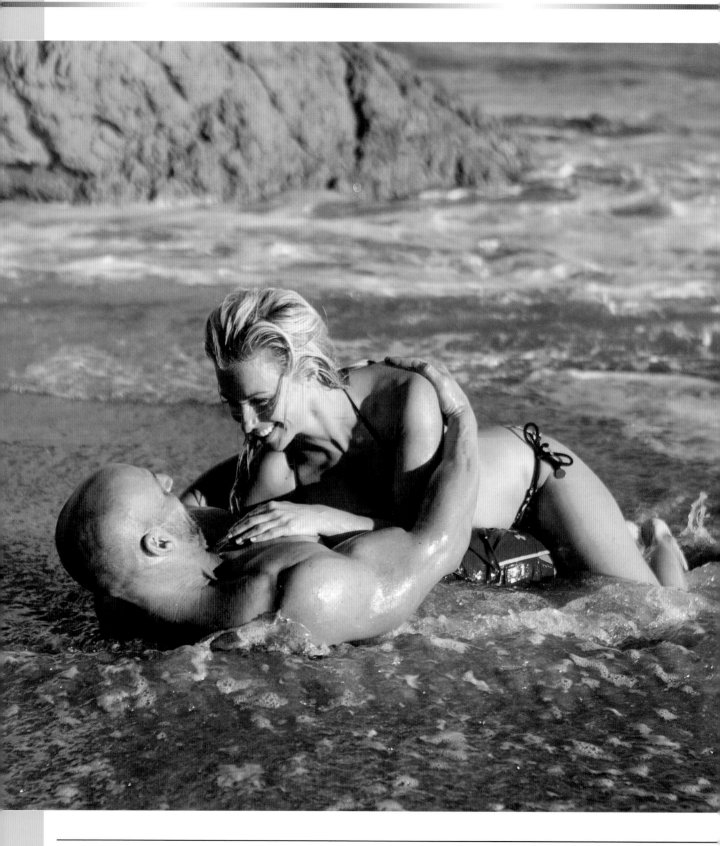

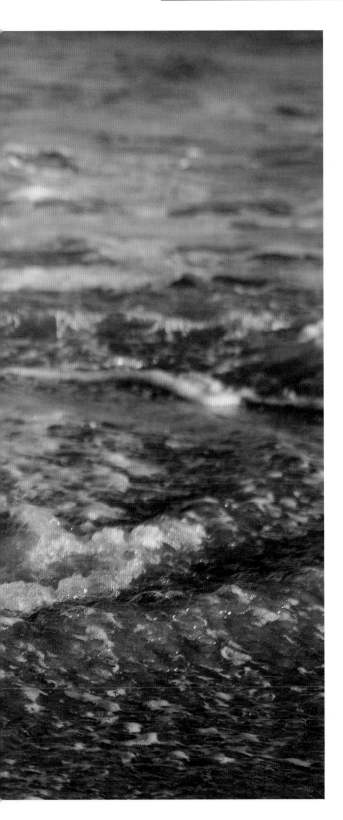

MAKE IT A COUPLE'S THING

Total-body transformation is an individual journey, but it doesn't mean you can't take someone else along for the ride. *Complete Physique* illustrates that working with a training partner is an effective strategy. Through both emotional and physical support, partners or couples work together, honing each other to be his or her best. The program itself is set up with tips on how to correctly spot each other during the exercises to garner the most out of each workout, and it features partner stretches that call for working together as a cohesive unit.

Whether two males, two females or a mixed pair, training with another person can be quite rewarding. You can both do your sets together, but the preferred way is for each to do a set followed by the other. This way you lend support, pushing your partner beyond a safe comfort zone and into the realm of new possibilities. Even if one partner is noticeably stronger than the other, you can make it a friendly "competition," each of you trying to best the other for reps. Perhaps partner A was able to complete eight reps on a target set. A goal for partner B might be to successfully get nine, despite lifting a lighter weight.

When working on machines, it's a simple pull of the pin to select the appropriate weight for differing levels of strength. With free weights, you can each take a side of the bar to freely slip on and off plates. Although you may want to perform your set immediately after you spot your partner's, it's best to rest long enough before starting so that you can give your all to your next set. Without ample rest, early and immediate failure is imminent.

Another benefit of training with a partner is that your partner can see and correct bad or inconsistent form that you or the mirror may not otherwise spot (pun intended). Perhaps you're pushing through your toes instead of your heels during a leg press. You can immediately correct yourself under the mindful and caring eye of your partner.

Training with someone who has a strength over your weakness will push you farther than you would have otherwise pushed yourself. It's also satisfying to see your partner getting stronger or past a sticking point on a certain exercise. Maybe your partner's balance has improved during lunges. Maybe you're finally able to complete a pull-up. When you later sit down to examine each other's before and after pics, it's a lot of fun and highly rewarding to see and point out just how far each of you has come.

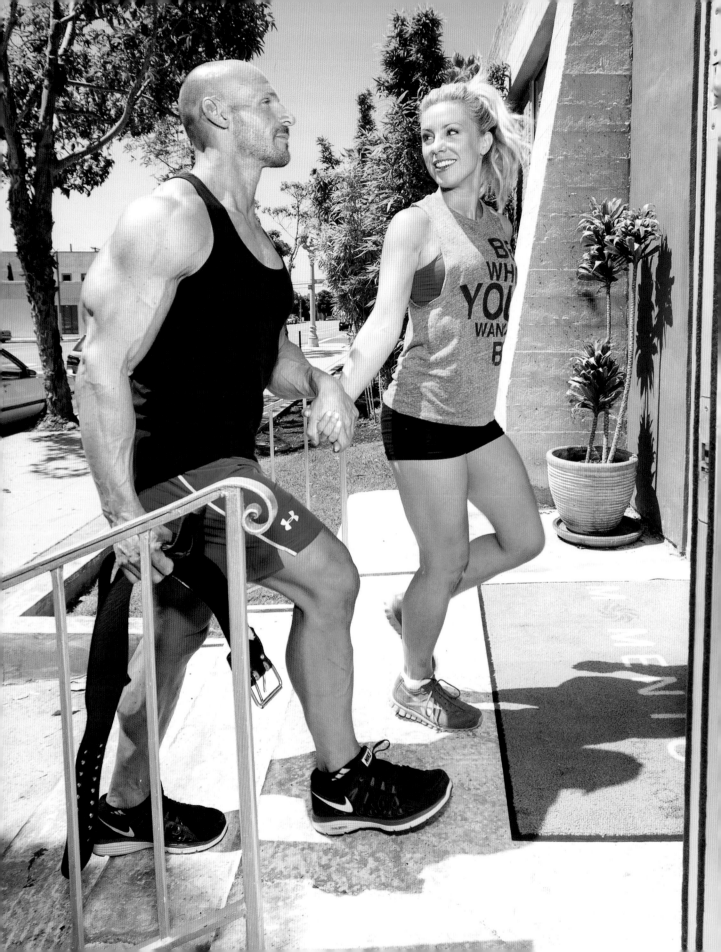

6 GYM WORKOUTS

The only thing random about your workouts should be the music. Have a plan—get results.

This is your *Complete Physique* gym workout plan. Although the regimen builds in intensity over its 12-week, three-phase time frame, results are not contingent on simply doing more. In later phases, as your strength and abilities increase, you will add increasingly challenging exercises, but tacking on more of them just for the sake of doing more is neither the goal nor the process. Think *better*, not *more*.

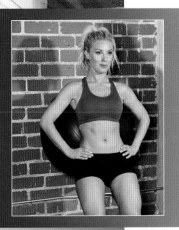
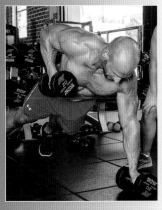
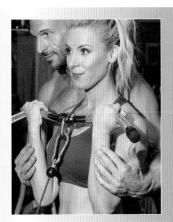
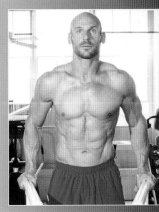

THE WORKOUTS

The following lists outline the three phases of the *Complete Physique* gym training protocol, detailing which exercises to perform and on which day. During each phase, each day of the week will be either a rest day or a workout day. For each workout day, the target areas are listed, along with the recommended cardio duration and stretch sequence. Next, you will find a list of exercises. Each exercise has corresponding numbers next to it indicating the total number of sets and repetitions you should perform. For example, "Smith Machine Shoulder Press 3X 8–12" translates to "three sets of 8 to 12 repetitions." Abdominal work is listed as a superset; for example "Reverse Crunch *superset with* Twisting Crunch 2X 15–20" translates to "both exercises performed back to back for two sets of 15 to 20 repetitions of each exercise."

Put your belief and efforts in yourself, because no one will ever care as much as you do. The hour or so of training per day is the time to be good to you—and your partner, if you work with one. Focus on firing or using the correct muscles during each set and repetition. If you're performing an Incline Dumbbell Press, for example, feel your chest doing the majority of the work with little help from your shoulders and triceps. Increase your target sets when you are able to do so and keep a record of them, and you absolutely will improve. "Is that all you got?" said no one ever, when they indeed gave all that they had.

PHASE 1: WEEKS 1–4
BEGINNER TRAINING PROTOCOL

MONDAY
Target: Back/abdominals
Cardio: 30 minutes
Exercises:
- Reverse-Grip Pulldown 3X 8–12
- Incline Dumbbell Row 3X 8–12
- Seated Cable Row 2X 8–12
- Sumo Deadlift *or* Kettlebell Sumo Deadlift 2X 8–10
- Reverse Crunch *superset with* Twisting Crunch 2X 15–20

Stretches:
- Partner Surrender Stretch
- Lower-Back Stretch

TUESDAY
Target: Chest/biceps

Cardio: 30 minutes
Exercises:
- Incline Dumbbell Press 3X 8–12
- Smith Machine Flat Press 3X 8–12
- Incline Dumbbell Flye 2X 12–15
- Low Pulley Flye 2X 12–15
- Reverse Barbell Curl 2X 10–12
- Cable Curl 2X 12–15
- Concentration Curl 2X 12–15 *per arm*

Stretches:
- Chest Stretch
- Biceps Stretch

WEDNESDAY: OFF

THURSDAY
Target: Legs
Cardio: None
Exercises:
- Swiss Ball Wall Squat 3X 12–15
- Single-Leg Press 2X 12–15 *per leg*
- Single-Leg Extension 2X 12–15 *per leg*
- Dumbbell Stiff-Legged Deadlift *or* Kettlebell Stiff-Legged Deadlift 3X 12–15
- Swiss Ball Hamstring Raise 2X 12–15
- Seated Calf Raise 3X 12–15

Stretches:
- Quad Stretch
- Glute/Groin Stretch
- Hamstrings Stretch
- Calf Stretch

FRIDAY
Target: Shoulders/triceps/abdominals
Cardio: 30 minutes
Exercises:
- Smith Machine Shoulder Press 3X 8–12
- Cable Lateral Raise 2X 10–12
- Bench Rear Lateral Raise 2X 10–12
- Dumbbell Upright Row 2X 10–12
- Lying Dumbbell Extension 2X 10–12
- Overhead Rope Extension 2X 10–12
- Reverse-Grip Pushdown 2X 10–15
- Reverse Crunch *superset with* Twisting Crunch 2X 15–20

Stretches:
- Deltoid Stretch
- Neck Stretch
- Triceps Stretch

SATURDAY: OFF

SUNDAY: OFF

PHASE 2: WEEKS 5–8
INTERMEDIATE TRAINING PROTOCOL

MONDAY
Target: Back/Abdominals
Cardio: 30 minutes
Exercises:
- Neutral-Grip Pull-Up 2X 8–10
- Reverse-Grip Pulldown 2X 8–12
- Incline Dumbbell Row 3X 8–12
- Seated Cable Row 2X 8–12
- Barbell Pullover or Machine Pullover 2X 8–12
- Sumo Deadlift or Kettlebell Sumo Deadlift 2X 8–10
- Reverse Crunch superset with Twisting Crunch 2X 15–20

Stretches:
- Partner Surrender Stretch
- Lower-Back Stretch

TUESDAY
Target: Chest/Biceps
Cardio: 30 minutes
Exercises:
- Incline Dumbbell Press 3X 8–12
- Smith Machine Flat Press 3X 8–12
- Incline Dumbbell Flye 2X 12–15
- Low Pulley Flye 2X 12–15
- Decline Push-Up or Bent-Knee Push-Up 2X 12–15
- Reverse Barbell Curl 2X 10–12
- Cable Curl 2X 12–15
- Overhead Pulley Curl 2X 12–15
- Concentration Curl 2X 12–15 per arm

Stretches:
- Chest Stretch
- Biceps Stretch

WEDNESDAY: OFF

THURSDAY
Target: Legs/Abdominals
Cardio: 30 minutes
Exercises:
- Front Squat 3X 12–15
- Single-Leg Press 2X 12–15 per leg
- Bench Lunge 2X 12–15 per leg
- Single-Leg Extension 2X 12–15 per leg
- Dumbbell Stiff-Legged Deadlift or Kettlebell Stiff-Legged Deadlift 3X 12–15
- One-legged Swiss Ball Curl 2X 12–15 per leg

- One-Legged Swiss Ball Curl 2X 12–15 per leg
- Seated Calf Raise 3X 12–15
- Swiss Ball Rollout superset with Swiss Ball Hip Crossover 2X 15–20

Stretches:
- Quad Stretch
- Glute/Groin Stretch
- Hamstring Stretch
- Calf Stretch

FRIDAY
Target: Shoulders/Triceps/Abdominals
Cardio: 30 minutes
Exercises:
- Smith Machine Shoulder Press 3X 8–12
- Alternating Front Dumbbell Raise 2X 10–12
- Cable Lateral Raise 2X 10–12
- Bench Rear Lateral Raise 2X 10–12
- Dumbbell Upright Row 2X 10–12
- Lying Dumbbell Extension 2X 10–12
- Vertical Dip or Bench Dip 2X 10–12
- Overhead Rope Extension 2X 10–12
- Reverse-Grip Pushdown 2X 10–15
- Reverse Crunch superset with Twisting Crunch 2X 15–20

Stretches:
- Deltoid Stretch
- Neck Stretch
- Triceps Stretch

SATURDAY: OFF

SUNDAY: OFF

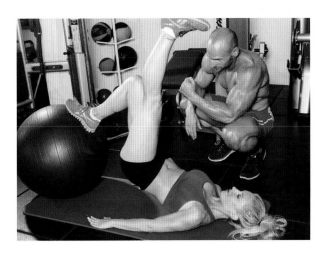

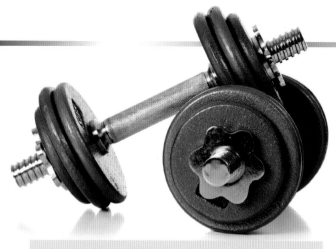

PHASE 3: WEEKS 9–12
ADVANCED TRAINING PROTOCOL

MONDAY
Target: Back/abdominals
Cardio: 40 minutes
Exercises:
- Neutral-Grip Pull-Up *or* Reverse-Grip Pull-Up 3X 8–10
- Reverse-Grip Barbell Row 2X 8–12
- Alternating Floor Row 2X 8–12 *per arm*
- Kettlebell One-Arm Row 2X 8–12 *per arm*
- Barbell Pullover or Machine Pullover 2X 8–12
- Sumo Deadlift *or* Kettlebell Sumo Deadlift 2X 8–10
- Hyperextension 2X 12–15
- Reverse Crunch *superset with* Twisting Crunch 2X 15–20

Stretches:
- Partner Surrender Stretch
- Lower-Back Stretch

TUESDAY
Target: Chest/biceps/abdominals
Cardio: 40 minutes
Exercises:
- Incline Dumbbell Press 3X 8–12
- Smith Machine Flat Press 3X 8–12
- Incline Dumbbell Flye 2X 12–15
- Low Pulley Flye 2X 12–15
- Decline Push-up 2X 12–15
- Reverse Barbell Curl 2X 10–12
- Cable Curl 2X 12–15
- Overhead Pulley Curl 2X 12–15
- Concentration Curl 2X 12–15 *per arm*
- Swiss Ball Rollout *superset with* Swiss Ball Hip Crossover 2X 15–20

Stretches:
- Chest Stretch
- Biceps Stretch

WEDNESDAY: OFF

THURSDAY
Target: Legs/abdominals
Cardio: 40 minutes
Exercises:
- Front Squat 3X 12–15
- Single-Leg Press 2X 12–15 *per leg*
- Bench Lunge 2X 12–15 *per leg*
- Single-Leg Extension 2X 12–15 *per leg*
- Dumbbell Stiff-Legged Deadlift *or* Kettlebell Stiff-Legged Deadlift 3X 12–15
- Swiss Ball Hamstring Raise 2X 12–15
- One-Legged Swiss Ball Curl 2X 12–15 *per leg*
- Seated Calf Raise 3X 12–15
- Swiss Ball Rollout *superset with* Swiss Ball Hip Crossover 2X 15–20

Stretches:
- Quad Stretch
- Glute/Groin Stretch
- Hamstrings Stretch
- Calf Stretch

FRIDAY
Target: Shoulders/triceps/abdominals
Cardio: 40 minutes
Exercises:
- Smith Machine Shoulder Press 3X 8–12 or Kettlebell One-Arm Clean and Press 3X 8–12 *per arm*
- Prone Shoulder Press 2X 10–12
- Cable Lateral Raise 2X 10–12
- Bench Rear Lateral Raise 2X 10–12
- Dumbbell Upright Row 2X 10–12
- Lying Dumbbell Extension 2X 10–12
- Vertical Dip *or* Bench Dip 2X 10–12
- Overhead Rope Extension 2X 10–12
- Reverse-Grip Pushdown 2X 10–15
- Reverse Crunch *superset with* Twisting Crunch 2X 15–20

Stretches:
- Deltoid Stretch
- Neck Stretch
- Triceps Stretch

SATURDAY
Cardio: 40 minutes

SUNDAY: OFF

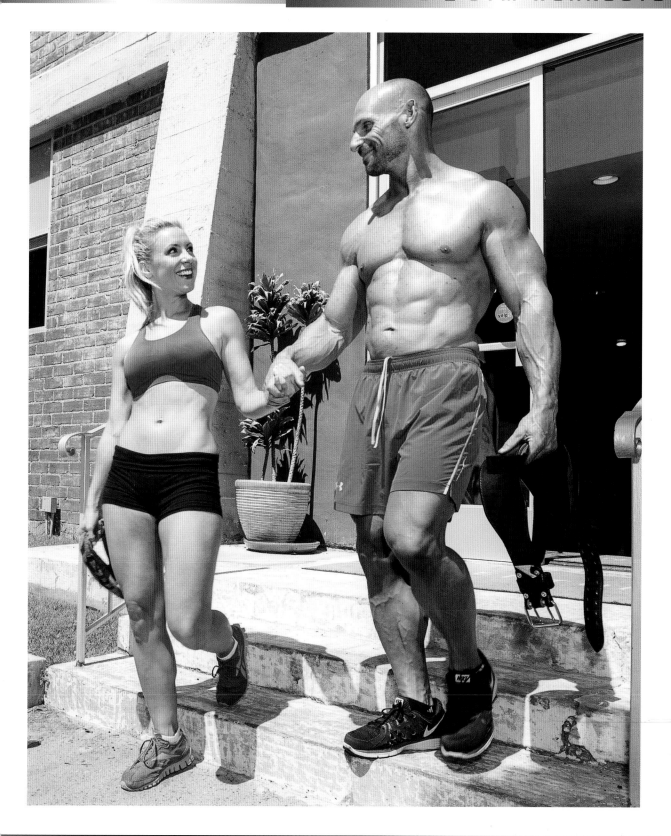

REVERSE-GRIP PULLDOWN

1 Sit with your thighs under the rollers of a lat pulldown machine while employing a close underhand grip on the bar.

2 Pull the bar down and backward until it touches your upper chest.

3 Return to the starting position with a full extension, and repeat for 8 to 12 repetitions.

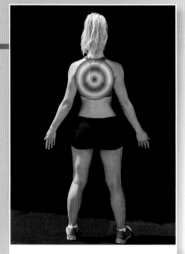

MUSCLE ACTION
Primary
- latissimus dorsi

Ancillary
- trapezius
- biceps brachii
- rhomboids
- forearm extensors
- forearm flexors

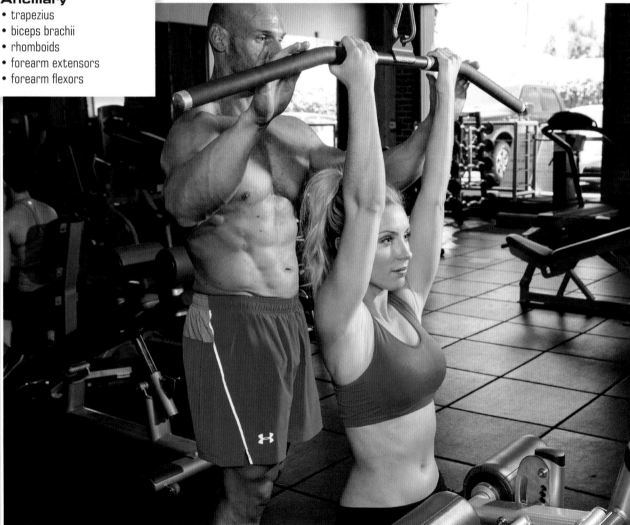

PROPER FORM
Do it right
- Look for a full stretch upward and a full contraction downward.
- Maintain an upright posture throughout.
- Lower your shoulders during the completion of the movement.

Avoid
- Leaning too far back and overusing your lower back.
- An incomplete range of motion.
- Using too much biceps to drive the movement.

MODIFICATIONS
Beginner
- A wider grip will decrease the range of motion.

Advanced
- Use an overhand grip.

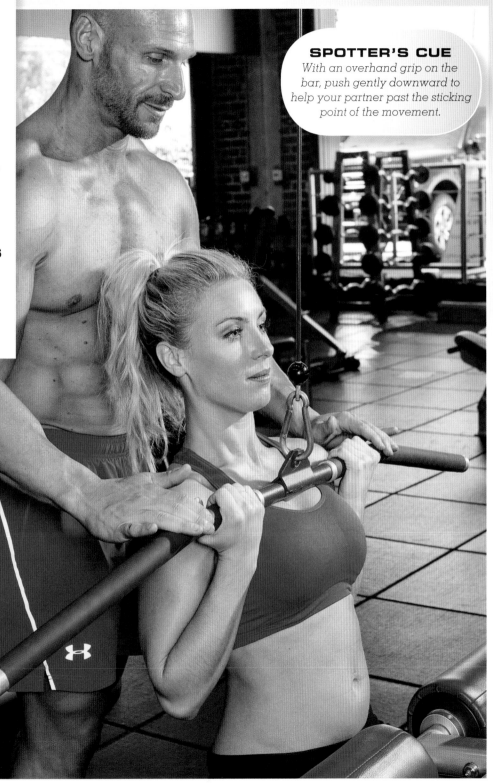

SPOTTER'S CUE
With an overhand grip on the bar, push gently downward to help your partner past the sticking point of the movement.

NEUTRAL-GRIP PULL-UP

1 Stand under a pull-up bar and grasp the bar with a neutral grip (palms facing each other). Bending your legs behind you, hang with your arms and shoulders fully extended.

2 Squeeze your shoulder blades and drive your elbows down to pull your chest toward the bar until it nearly touches it.

3 Lower to a full stretch, and then repeat for 8 to 10 repetitions.

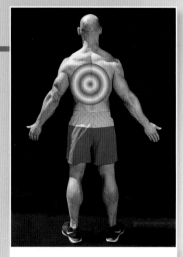

MUSCLE ACTION
Primary
- latissimus dorsi

Ancillary
- trapezius
- biceps brachii
- rhomboids
- forearm extensors
- forearm flexors

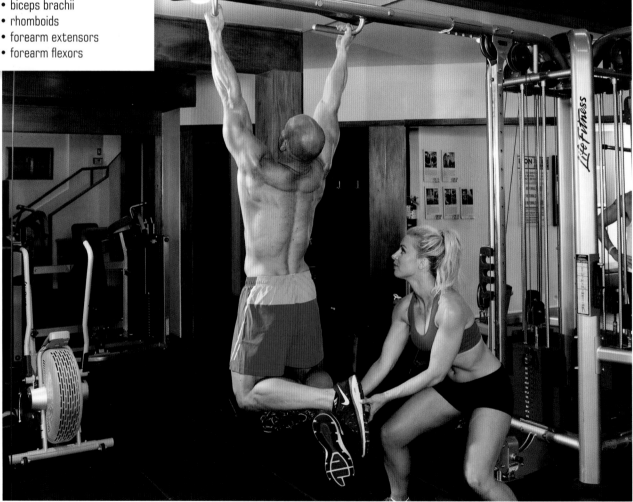

PROPER FORM
Do it right
- Look for a full stretch downward and a full contraction at the top.
- Keep your chest up and shoulders back.
- Use your lats to drive the movement.

Avoid
- Leaning too far back and overusing your lower back.
- An incomplete range of motion.
- Using too much biceps to drive the movement.

MODIFICATIONS
Beginner
- A wider grip will decrease the range of motion.

Advanced
- Use an overhand grip.

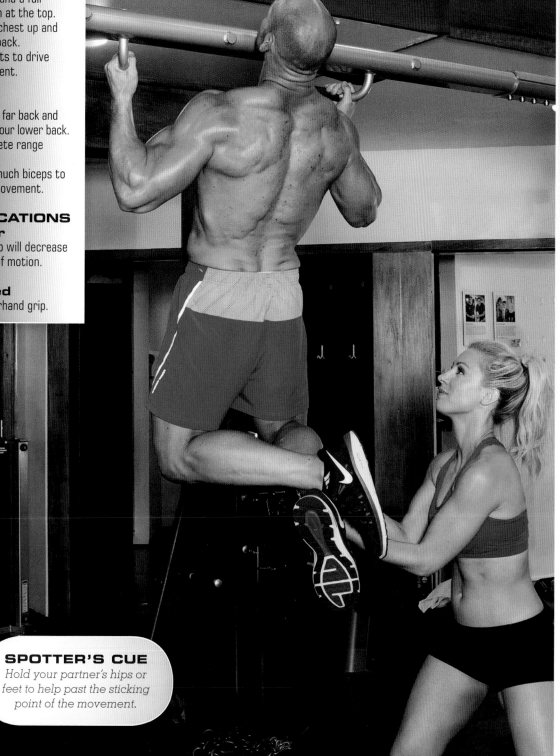

SPOTTER'S CUE
Hold your partner's hips or feet to help past the sticking point of the movement.

REVERSE-GRIP PULL-UP

1 Stand under a pull-up bar and grasp the bar with a close underhand grip, palms facing you. Bending your legs behind you, hang with your arms and shoulders fully extended.

2 Pull your chest toward the bar until it nearly touches it.

3 Lower to a full stretch, and then repeat for 8 to 10 repetitions.

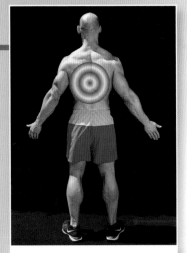

MUSCLE ACTION
Primary
- latissimus dorsi

Ancillary
- trapezius
- biceps brachii
- rhomboids
- forearm extensors
- forearm flexors

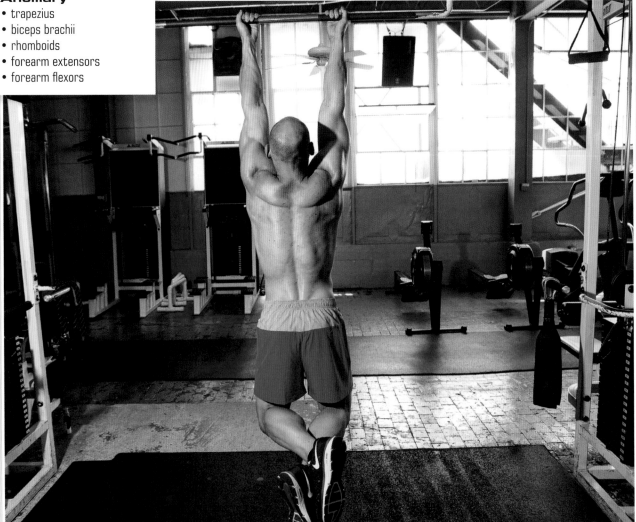

PROPER FORM
Do it right
- Look for a full stretch downward and a full contraction at the top.
- Keep your chest up.
- Use your lats to drive the movement.

Avoid
- Leaning too far back and overusing your lower back.
- An incomplete range of motion.
- Using too much biceps to drive the movement.

MODIFICATIONS
Beginner
- A wider grip will decrease the range of motion.

Advanced
- Use an overhand grip.

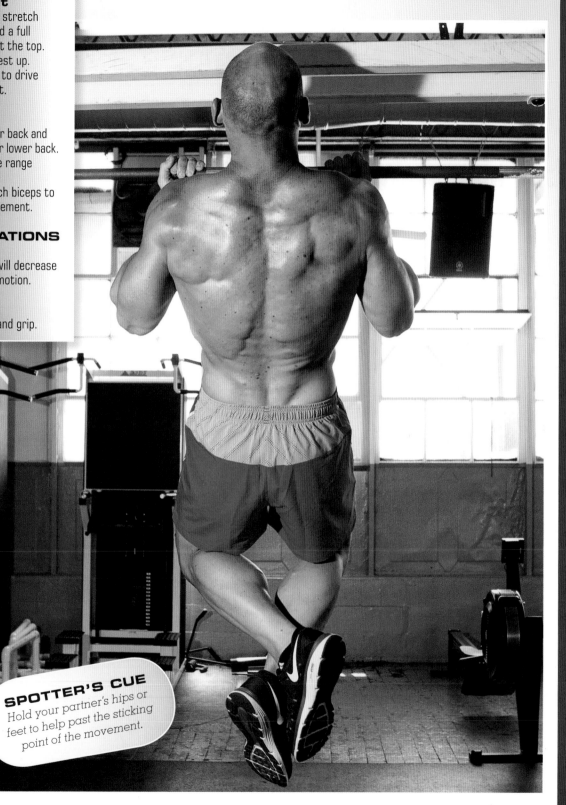

SPOTTER'S CUE
Hold your partner's hips or feet to help past the sticking point of the movement.

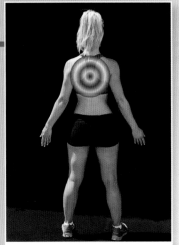

INCLINE DUMBBELL ROW

1 Lie facedown on an incline bench with your chest against the pad and your legs bent and positioned on the pads. With your palms facing inward, grab a dumbbell with each hand letting them hang straight down so that your arms are fully extended.

2 While keeping your elbows in, pull the dumbbells upward and back until they nearly touch your chest.

3 Lower, and repeat for 8 to 12 repetitions.

MUSCLE ACTION
Primary
- latissimus dorsi
- trapezius
- rhomboids

Ancillary
- biceps brachii
- rear deltoids
- erector spinae
- forearm extensors
- forearm flexors

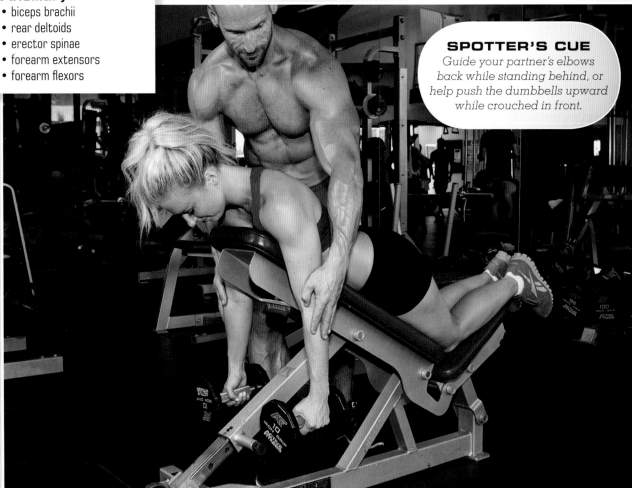

SPOTTER'S CUE
Guide your partner's elbows back while standing behind, or help push the dumbbells upward while crouched in front.

PROPER FORM
Do it right
- Look for a full stretch downward and a full contraction at the top.
- Maintain a flat back throughout.
- Use your lats to drive the movement.

Avoid
- Overarching and overusing your lower back.
- Allowing the dumbbells to drop too far forward.
- Using too much biceps to drive the movement.

MODIFICATIONS
Beginner
- Use a barbell.

Advanced
- Alternate arms.

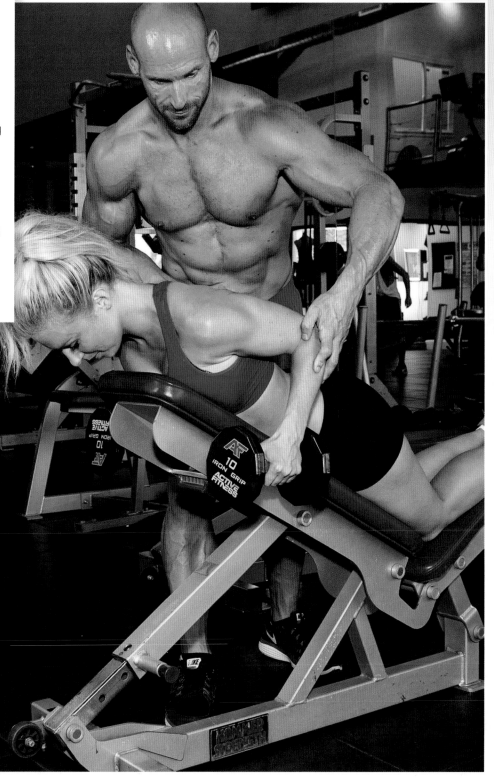

REVERSE-GRIP BARBELL ROW

1 Grasp a barbell with an underhand grip and your hands shoulder-width apart while standing with your knees bent slightly. Bend forward at the waist with a flat back, allowing the weight to hang straight down so that your arms are fully extended.

2 Pull the barbell upward and back until it nearly touches your navel.

3 Lower, and repeat for 8 to 12 repetitions.

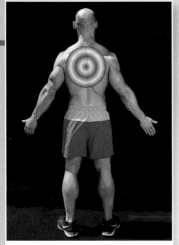

MUSCLE ACTION
Primary
- latissimus dorsi
- trapezius
- rhomboids

Ancillary
- biceps brachii
- rear deltoids
- erector spinae
- forearm extensors
- forearm flexors

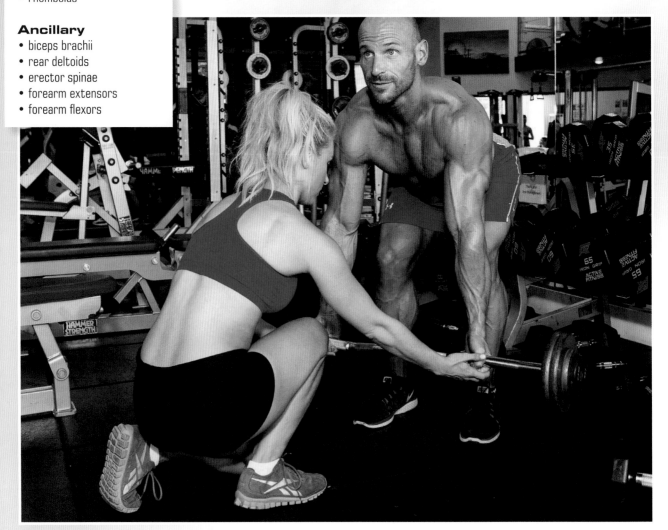

PROPER FORM
Do it right
- Look for a full stretch downward and a full contraction at the top.
- Maintain a flat back throughout.
- Pull both up and backward into your midriff.

Avoid
- Rounding your back.
- Excessively swinging the weight.
- Using too much biceps to drive the movement.

MODIFICATIONS
Beginner
- A wider grip will decrease the range of motion.

Advanced
- Use dumbbells.

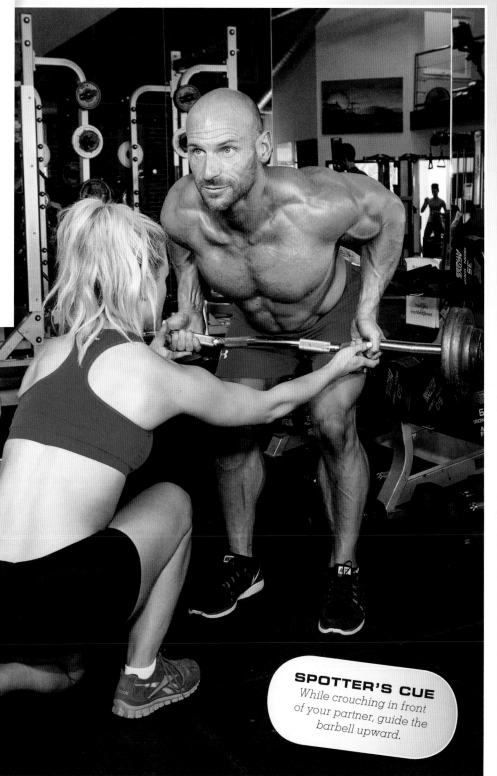

SPOTTER'S CUE
While crouching in front of your partner, guide the barbell upward.

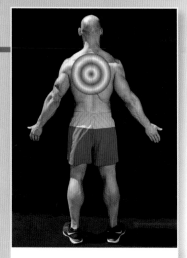

ALTERNATING FLOOR ROW

1 Place two flat-sided dumbbells on the floor about shoulder-width apart. Position yourself on your toes and your hands as if you were doing a push-up, with your body in a straight, plank-like position.

2 Pull one arm up and back toward your chest while keeping your torso stabilized.

3 Lower, and repeat with the other arm. Alternate sides for 8 to 12 repetitions per arm.

MUSCLE ACTION

Primary
- latissimus dorsi
- trapezius
- rhomboids

Ancillary
- biceps brachii
- rear deltoids
- rectus abdominis
- obliques
- erector spinae
- forearm extensors
- forearm flexors

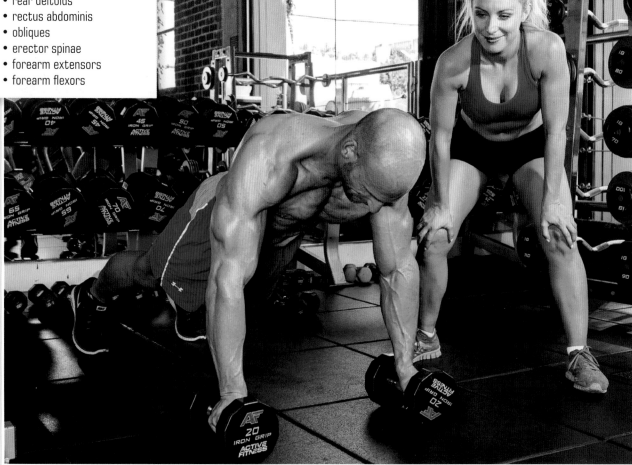

PROPER FORM
Do it right
- A full contraction at the top of the movement.
- Retract the shoulder blade of the working side as you flex your elbow to pull the weight upward.
- Maintain a stabilized torso throughout.

Avoid
- Dropping your torso.
- Raising your hips too high.
- Excessively jerking the weight.

MODIFICATIONS
Beginner
- Try it with bent legs.

Advanced
- Briefly hold the contracted portion of the movement.

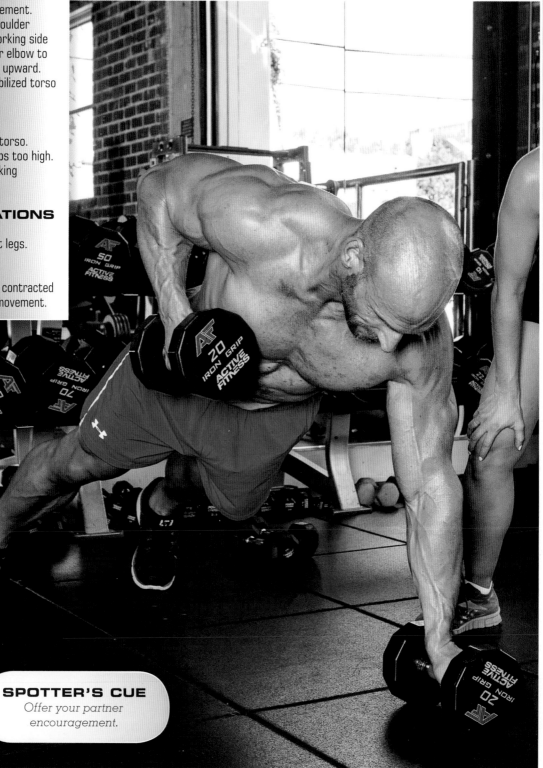

SPOTTER'S CUE
Offer your partner encouragement.

KETTLEBELL ONE-ARM ROW

1 Stand holding a kettlebell in one hand. Lean forward until your torso is parallel to the ground, while extending your free arm straight ahead and your opposite leg behind you.

2 Starting with the kettlebell dangling below, pull straight up until it nearly touches your chest.

3 Lower, and repeat for 8 to 12 repetitions per arm.

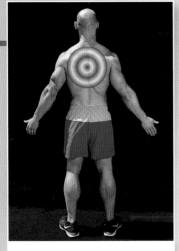

MUSCLE ACTION
Primary
- latissimus dorsi
- trapezius
- rhomboids

Ancillary
- biceps brachii
- rear deltoids
- rectus abdominis
- obliques
- erector spinae
- forearm extensors
- forearm flexors

SPOTTER'S CUE
Help your partner to maintain balance by holding the extended hand.

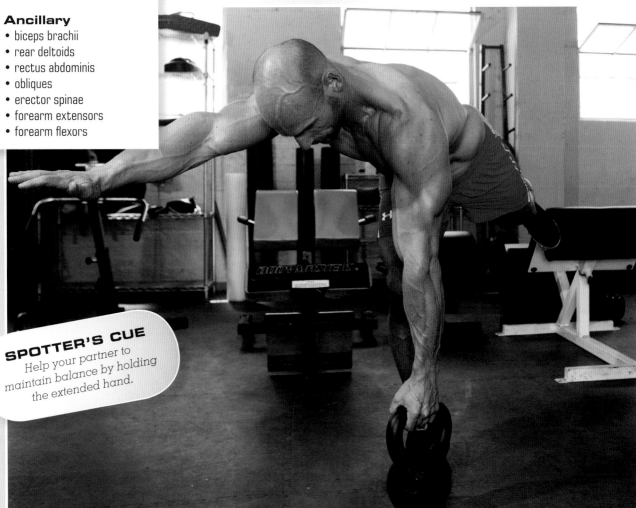

PROPER FORM
Do it right
- Look for a full contraction at the top.
- Maintain a stabilized torso throughout.
- Move through a fluid range of motion.

Avoid
- Dropping your extended leg or arm.
- Placing too much pressure on your toes.
- Excessively swinging the weight.

MODIFICATIONS
Beginner
- Firmly plant both feet.

Advanced
- Hold a barbell at its center.

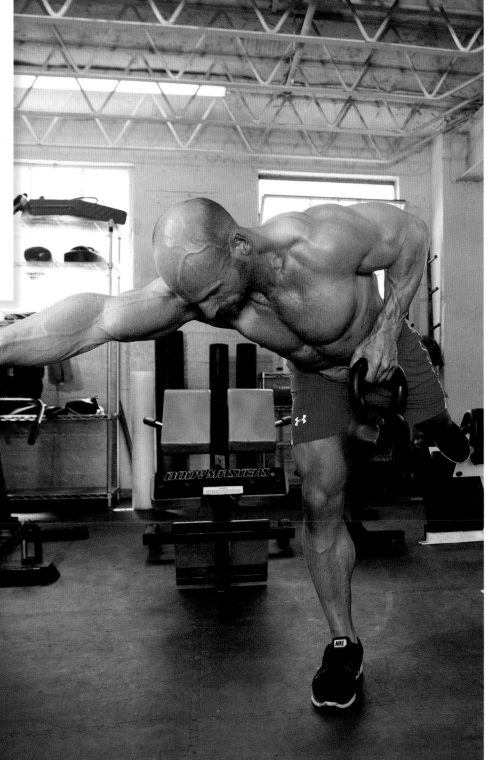

SEATED CABLE ROW

1 Sit with your legs bent and your feet placed on the pads of a cable row machine while holding the bar attachment with a neutral grip, your palms facing each other. Keeping your back flat, stretch forward, feeling the stretch in your lats.

2 Lean back while pulling the bar into your midriff, thrusting your chest forward and your shoulders back in the finished position.

3 Repeat for 8 to 12 repetitions.

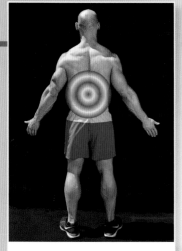

MUSCLE ACTION
Primary
- latissimus dorsi
- outer back
- erector spinae

Ancillary
- biceps brachii
- rear deltoids
- rectus abdominis
- forearm extensors
- forearm flexors

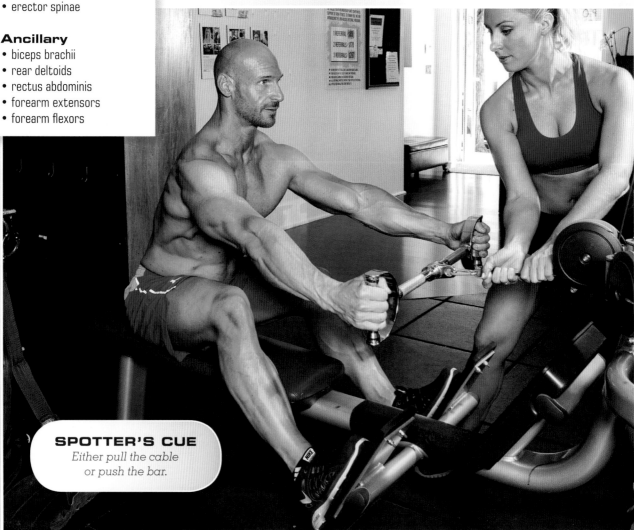

SPOTTER'S CUE
Either pull the cable or push the bar.

PROPER FORM
Do it right
- Perform a full stretch at the start of the movement.
- Thrust out your chest at the completion of the movement.
- Maintain a flat back throughout.

Avoid
- Rounding your back.
- Using too much biceps to drive the movement.
- Excessively swinging the weight.

MODIFICATIONS
Beginner
- Use a v-bar attachment.

Advanced
- Use one arm at a time with a single pulley.

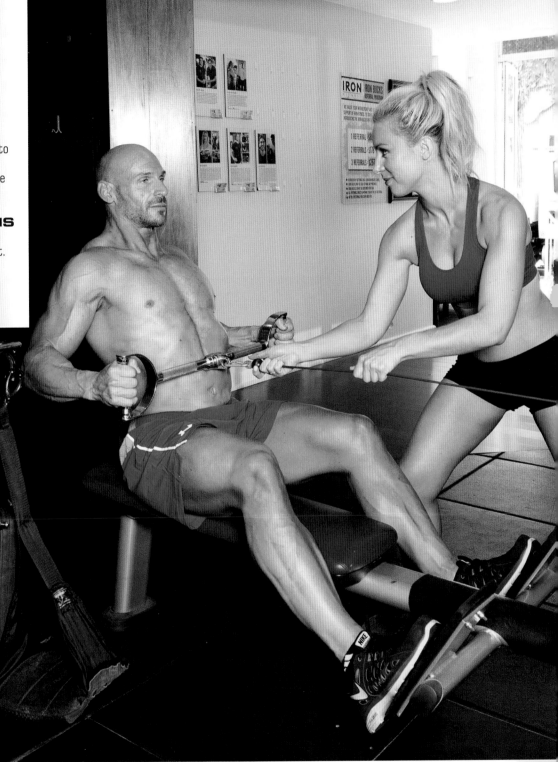

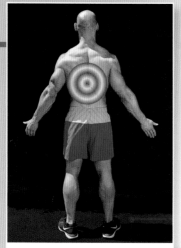

BARBELL PULLOVER

1 Lie on your back with your feet planted on either side of a flat bench as you hold a barbell with an overhand grip less than shoulder-width apart. Stretch your arms well behind your head, feeling the stretch in the lats.

2 Keeping your arms bent, bring the barbell over our head and then downward in an arc-like motiong until your hands rest just above your navel.

3 Return back to the starting position along the same pathway as you exhale for 8 to 12 repetitions.

MUSCLE ACTION
Primary
- latissimus dorsi
- serratus anterior

Ancillary
- deltoids
- triceps brachii
- rectus abdominis

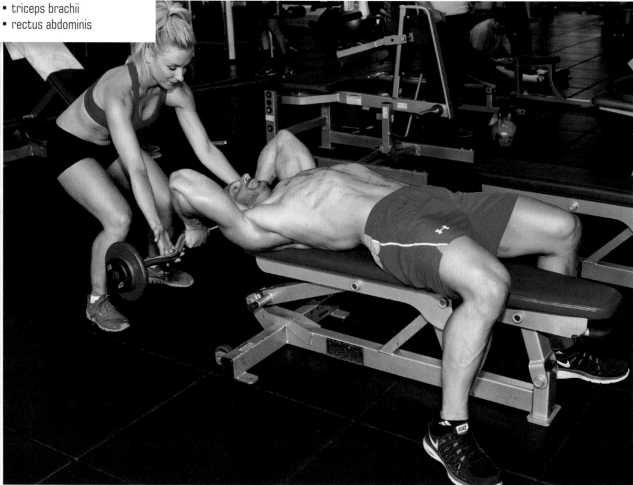

PROPER FORM
Do it right
- Lower the bar with control.
- Perform a full stretch behind your head.
- Maintain a flat back throughout.

Avoid
- Raising your lower back.
- Excessively stretching behind your head.
- Excessive speed.

MODIFICATIONS
Beginner
- Use a dumbbell.

Advanced
- Use a close underhand grip.

SPOTTER'S CUE
Help your partner by pushing upward on the bar.

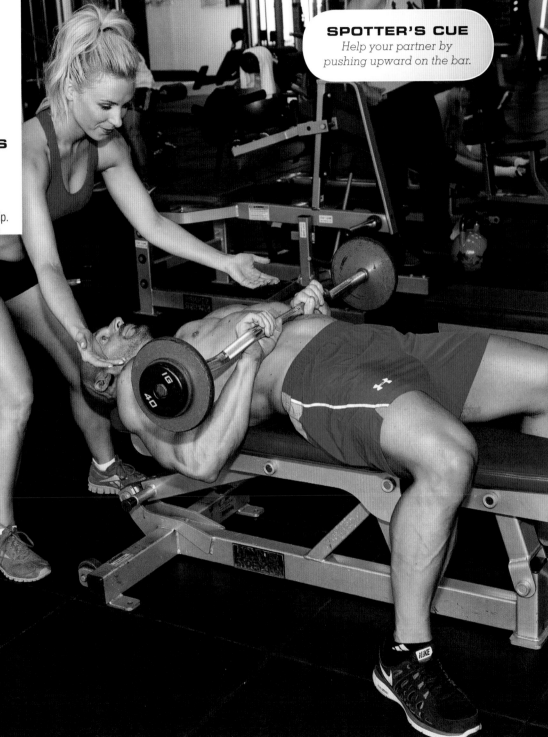

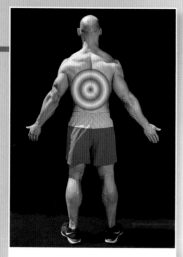

MUSCLE ACTION
Primary
- latissimus dorsi
- serratus anterior

Ancillary
- deltoids
- triceps brachii
- rectus abdominis

MACHINE PULLOVER

1 Begin seated in a pullover machine. Adjust the seat so that when your arms are raised overhead, your elbows will be centered on the elbow pads.

2 Step on the bar at your feet to bring the apparatus in front of you. Place your elbows on the pad, and grasp the bar with an overhand grip, and then step off the bar. Stretch your arms backward to the start position.

3 Drive your elbows down and back so that the bar moves toward your abdomen, contracting your lats as you move.

4 Stretch back, and perform 8 to 12 repetitions. When finished, use the foot bar to catch the weight, and then remove your arms and slowly let the weight return to its starting position.

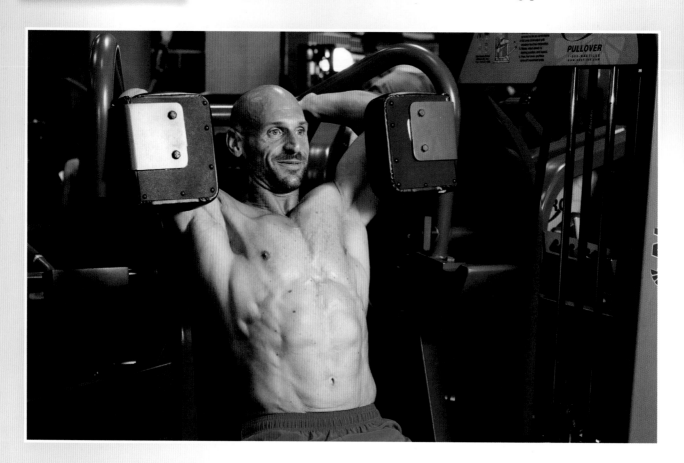

PROPER FORM
Do it right
- Lower the bar with control.
- Fully expand your chest.
- Keep your elbows firmly on the pads throughout the exercise.

Avoid
- Pulling away from the back pad.
- Excessively stretching behind your head.
- Releasing your arms from the bar before pushing the foot bar.

MODIFICATIONS
Beginner
- Use a lighter weight.

Advanced
- Use a close underhand grip.

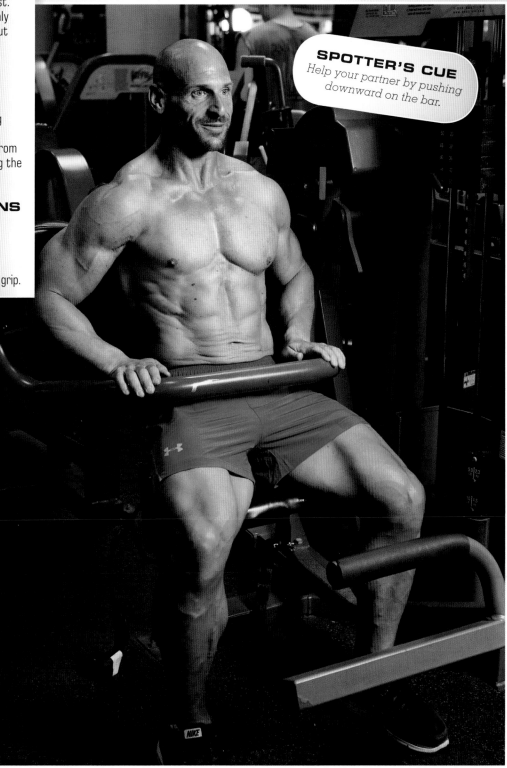

SPOTTER'S CUE
Help your partner by pushing downward on the bar.

SUMO DEADLIFT

1 Stand in front of a weighted barbell with your feet very wide apart and your toes facing angled outward. Squat down, and grab the barbell with an overhand grip, your wrists in line with your elbows. Your chest should be directly above the bar, your spine straight and your head up.

2 Push through your heels while maintaining a flat back as you stand upright until your arms are fully extended downward.

3 Carefully lower the barbell back to the ground, and repeat for 8 to 10 repetitions.

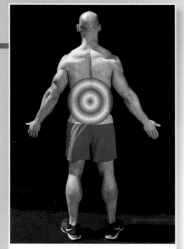

MUSCLE ACTION
Primary
- erector spinae
- hamstrings
- gluteus maximus
- rectus abdominis
- quadriceps

Ancillary
- trapezius
- biceps
- forearm extensors
- forearm flexors

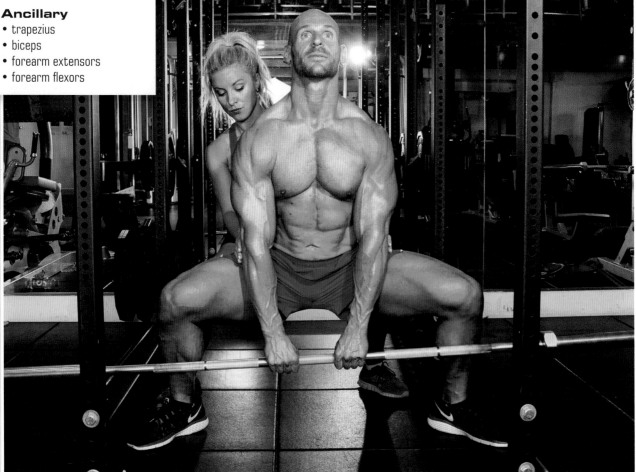

PROPER FORM
Do it right
- Push through your heels to drive the movement.
- Keep the bar close to your body.
- Stand completely erect at the top of the movement.

Avoid
- Rounding your back.
- Letting the weight drop.
- Pushing through your toes.

MODIFICATIONS
Beginner
- Use just the bar.

Advanced
- A closer stance will increase the range of motion.

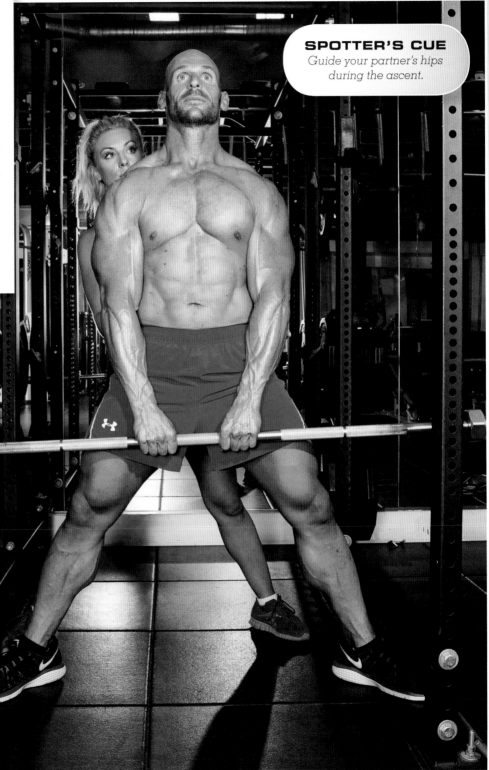

SPOTTER'S CUE
Guide your partner's hips during the ascent.

KETTLEBELL SUMO DEADLIFT

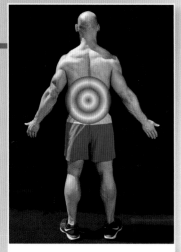

1 Grasping a kettlebell with a close, overhand grip, squat down with your legs spread apart and your toes angled outward.

2 Push through your heels while maintaining a flat back as you stand upright until your arms are fully extended downward.

3 Repeat for 8 to 10 repetitions.

MUSCLE ACTION
Primary
- erector spinae
- hamstrings
- gluteus maximus
- rectus abdominis
- quadriceps

Ancillary
- trapezius
- biceps
- forearm extensors
- forearm flexors

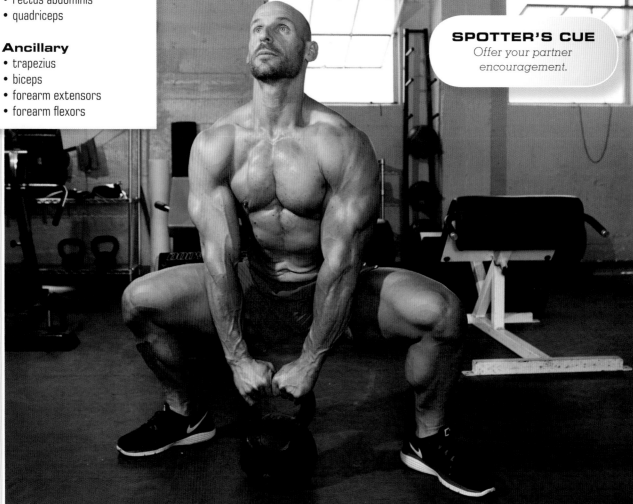

SPOTTER'S CUE
Offer your partner encouragement.

PROPER FORM
Do it right
- Push through your heels to drive the movement.
- Keep the kettlebell close to your body.
- Stand completely erect at the top of the movement.

Avoid
- Rounding your back.
- Letting the kettlebell drop.
- Pushing through your toes.

MODIFICATIONS
Beginner
- Use a lighter resistance.

Advanced
- A closer stance will increase the range of motion.

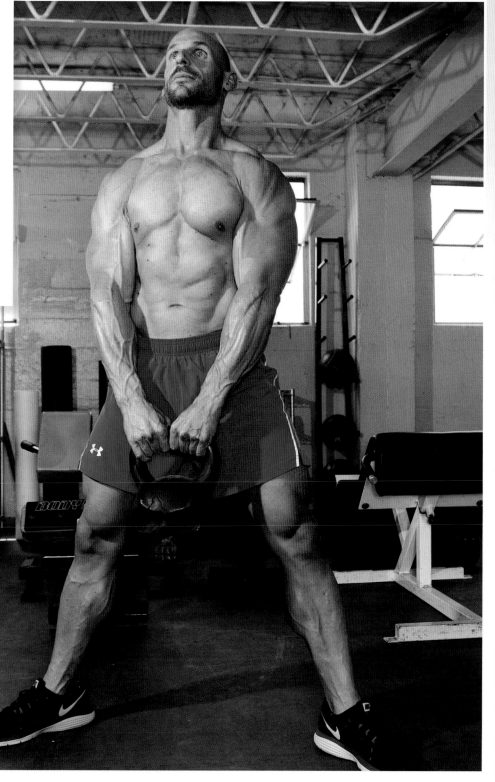

HYPEREXTENSION

1 Position yourself in a hyperextension bench with your lower legs pressed back against the pads and your arms folded across your chest with your torso bent downward at the waist.

2 Raise your torso until your entire body is one straight line and parallel to the ground.

3 Lower your torso, and then repeat for 12 to 15 repetitions.

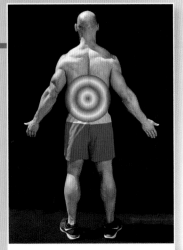

MUSCLE ACTION
Primary
- erector spinae

Ancillary
- gluteus maximus
- hamstrings

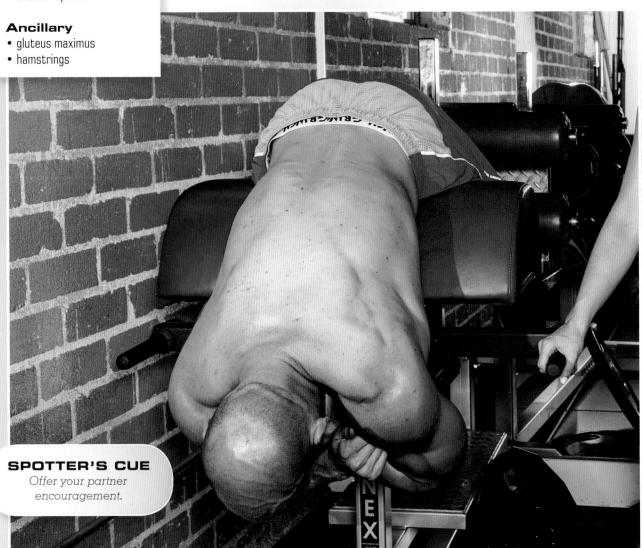

SPOTTER'S CUE
*Offer your partner
encouragement.*

PROPER FORM
Do it right
- Raise your body smoothly and with control.
- Keep your body in one straight line at the top of the movement.
- Contract your core at the top of each repetition.

Avoid
- Lifting your torso too high.
- Excessive swinging.
- Pressing your pelvis too hard against the pad.

MODIFICATIONS
Beginner
- Perform fewer repetitions.

Advanced
- Hold a barbell plate across your chest for added resistance.

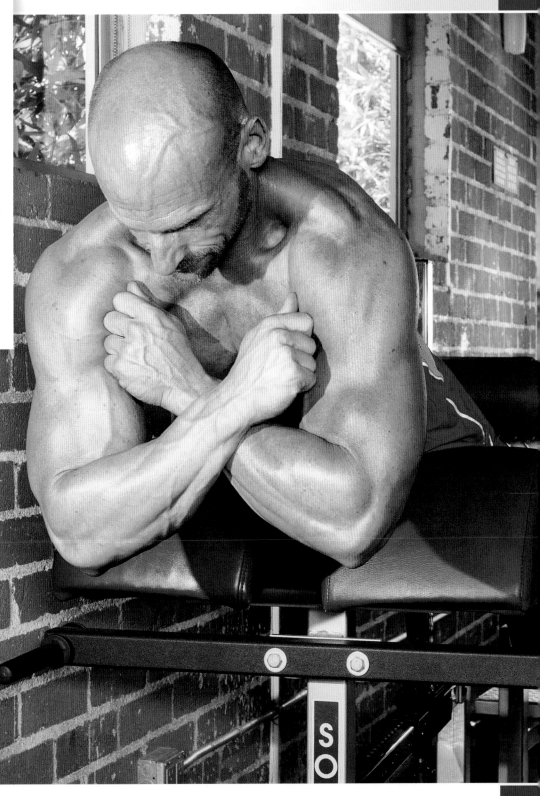

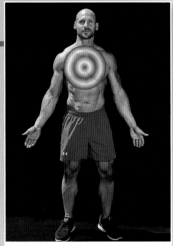

INCLINE DUMBBELL PRESS

1 Lie back on an incline press with your feet planted on the ground and a pair of dumbbells positioned next to your outer shoulders.

2 Push upward over your chest and arc inward so the dumbbells are nearly touching at the locked-out position with your arms fully extended upward.

3 Lower along the same pathway, and repeat for 8 to 12 repetitions.

MUSCLE ACTION
Primary
- pectoralis major

Ancillary
- anterior deltoids
- triceps brachii
- rectus abdominis
- erector spinae

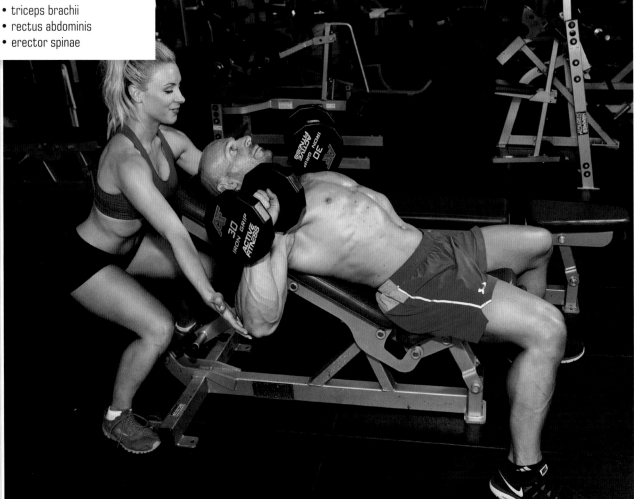

PROPER FORM
Do it right
- Use a controlled descent.
- Bring the dumbbells to your outer shoulders.
- Keep your feet planted on the ground.

Avoid
- Arching your back.
- Bouncing the dumbbells off your chest.
- Excessive speed.

MODIFICATIONS
Beginner
- Reduce the angle of incline.

Advanced
- Alternate arms.

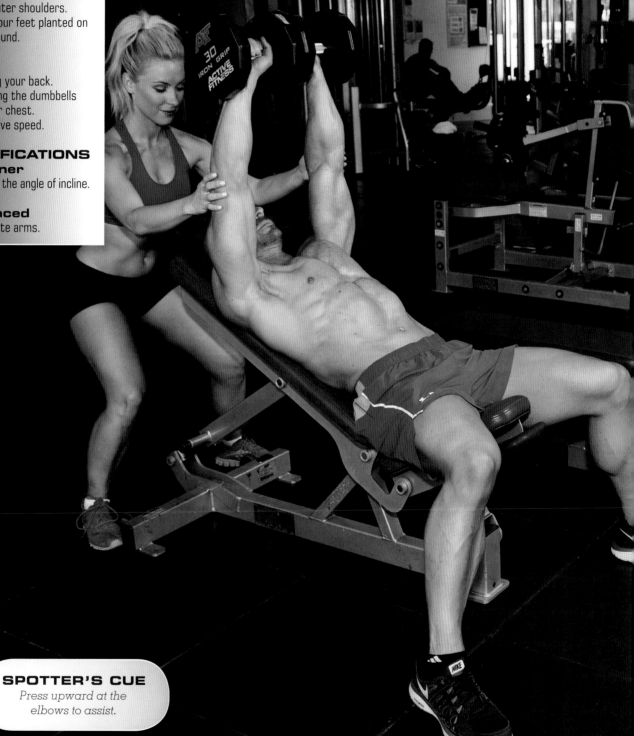

SPOTTER'S CUE
Press upward at the elbows to assist.

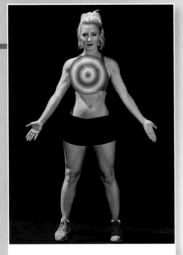

SMITH MACHINE FLAT PRESS

1 Lie back on a flat bench under a Smith machine with your feet planted on the ground and the bar directly above your chest.

2 Unrack the bar, and lower it to your chest while keeping your elbows flared out.

3 Leading with your chest, push straight up to full lockout with your arms fully extended, and repeat for 8 to 12 repetitions.

MUSCLE ACTION
Primary
- pectoralis major

Ancillary
- anterior deltoids
- triceps brachii
- rectus abdominis
- erector spinae

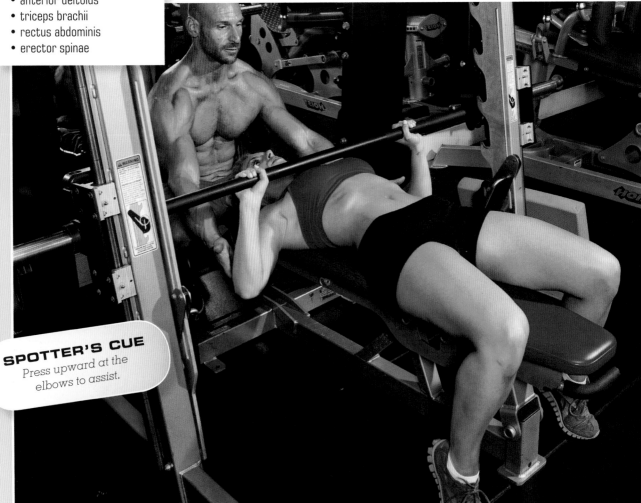

SPOTTER'S CUE
Press upward at the elbows to assist.

PROPER FORM
Do it right
- Use a controlled descent.
- Lower the barbell to your nipple line.
- Keep your feet planted on the ground.

Avoid
- Arching your back.
- Bouncing the bar off your chest.
- Excessive speed.

MODIFICATIONS
Beginner
- A wider grip will decrease the range of motion.

Advanced
- A closer grip will increase the range of motion.

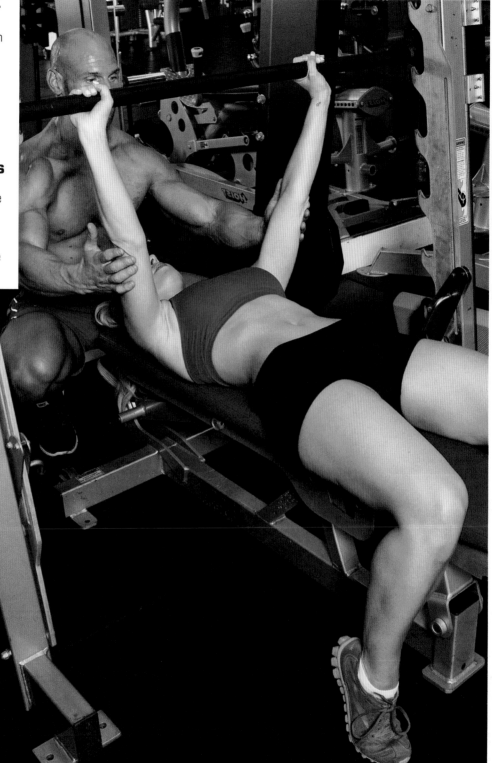

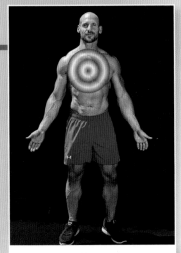

INCLINE DUMBBELL FLYE

1 Lie back on an incline press with your feet planted on the ground and hold a pair of dumbbells with your palms facing each other. Bend your arms as you stretch them out to your sides, feeling the stretch in your chest.

2 Push your chest muscles together as you straighten your arms upward as you arc in along the same pathway, finishing with your arms directly over your chest with your elbows locked.

3 Lower the dumbells along the same pathway, and repeat for 12 to 15 repetitions.

MUSCLE ACTION
Primary
• pectoralis major

Ancillary
• anterior deltoids
• rectus abdominis
• erector spinae

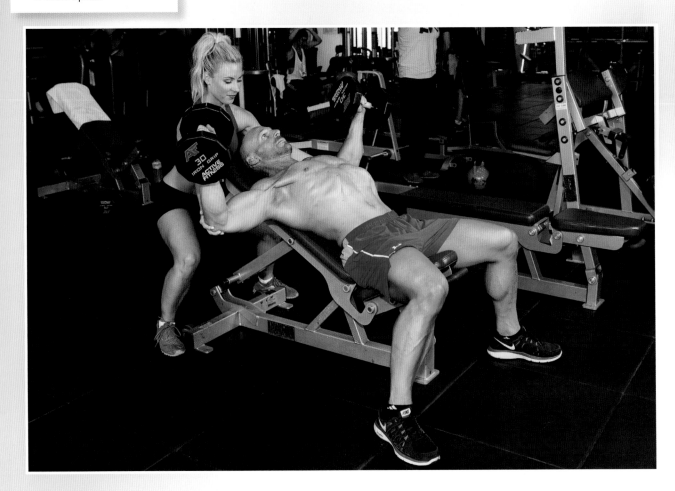

PROPER FORM
Do it right
- Lower the dumbbells with control.
- Squeeze your pecs together at the top of the movement.
- Keep your elbows slightly bent as you move your arms outward.

Avoid
- Arching your back.
- Straightening your arms out to your sides.
- Excessive speed.

MODIFICATIONS
Beginner
- Use a lighter weight.

Advanced
- Alternate arms.

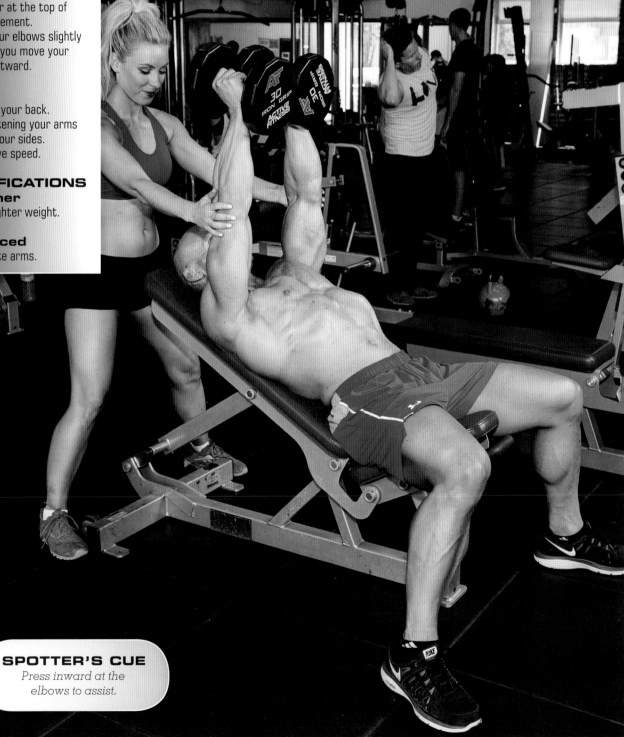

SPOTTER'S CUE
Press inward at the elbows to assist.

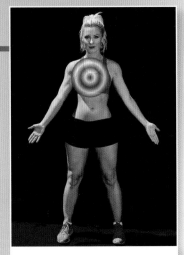

LOW PULLEY FLYE

1 Stand in the middle of a cable stack with a pair of handles attached at the lower cable attachments. With a staggered stance, grasp a handle in each hand.

2 With your elbows slightly bent, bring your arms forward in a scooping motion, finishing with both arms well in front of your chest and squeezing them together.

3 Lower along the same pathway for 12 to 15 repetitions.

MUSCLE ACTION
Primary
- pectoralis major

Ancillary
- anterior deltoids
- rectus abdominis
- erector spinae

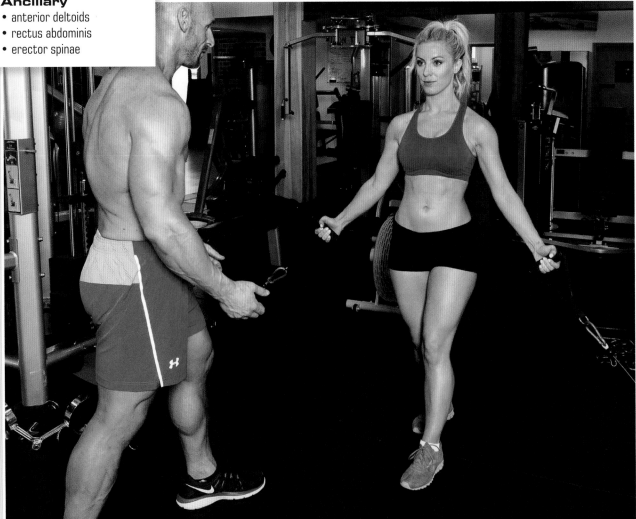

PROPER FORM
Do it right
- Keep your arms slightly bent throughout.
- Lift both upward and away from your body.
- Maintain a staggered stance throughout.

Avoid
- Arching your back.
- Using too much biceps to drive the movement.
- Raising your arms higher than chest level.

MODIFICATIONS
Beginner
- Use a lighter weight.

Advanced
- Alternate arms.

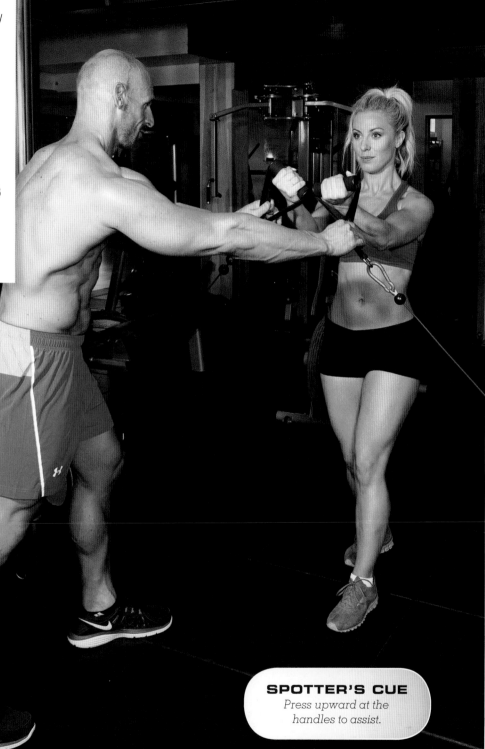

SPOTTER'S CUE
Press upward at the handles to assist.

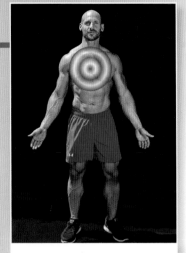

DECLINE PUSH-UP

1 Position your toes on a bench and your body in an elongated, decline position with your hands placed on the floor shoulder-width apart.

2 Lower your chest nearly to the ground by bending at the elbows while keeping your chest directly above your hands. Repeat for 12 to 15 repetitions.

MUSCLE ACTION
Primary
- pectoralis major

Ancillary
- anterior deltoids
- rhomboids
- triceps brachii
- rectus abdominis
- erector spinae

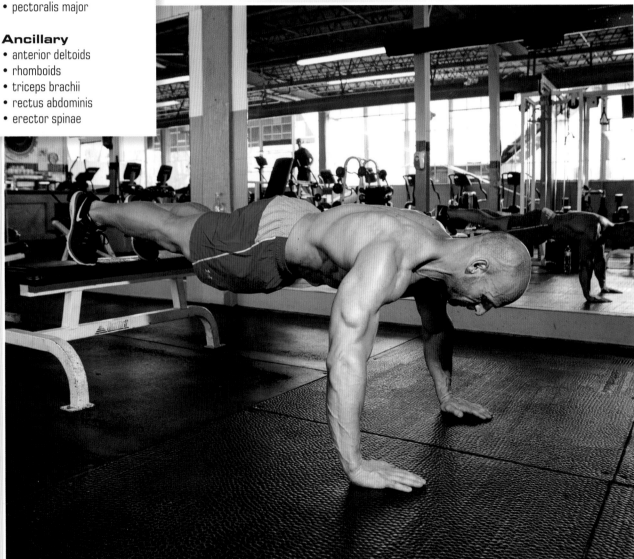

PROPER FORM
Do it right
- Perform slow and controlled repetitions.
- Keep your upper body straight and stabilize your torso throughout.
- Lower yourself until your upper arms are parallel to the ground.

Avoid
- Excessive speed.
- Shallow or bouncy repetitions.
- Allowing your lower back to dip too far.

MODIFICATIONS
Beginner
- A wider hand spacing will decrease the range of motion.

Advanced
- Raise one leg.

SPOTTER'S CUE
You can help by raising your partner's hips.

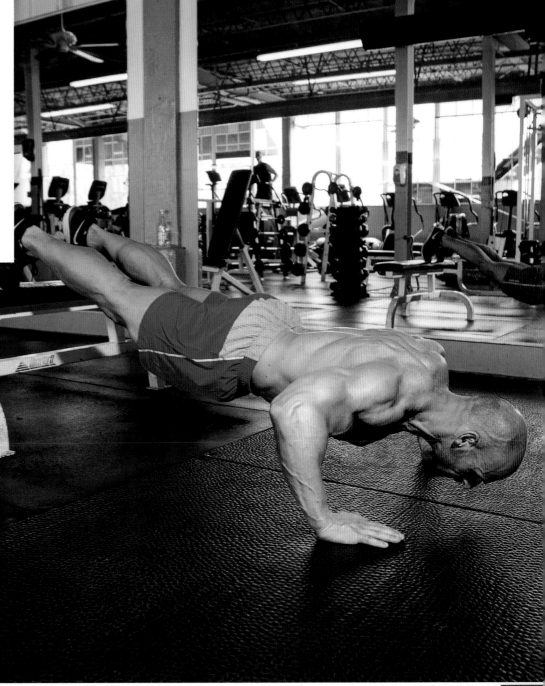

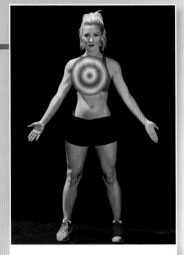

BENT-KNEE PUSH-UP

1 With your knees on the ground and your body in an elongated position, place your hands on the floor shoulder-width apart.

2 Lower your chest nearly to the ground by bending at the elbows while keeping your chest directly above your hands. Repeat for 12 to 15 repetitions.

MUSCLE ACTION
Primary
- pectoralis major

Ancillary
- anterior deltoids
- rhomboids
- triceps brachii
- rectus abdominis
- erector spinae

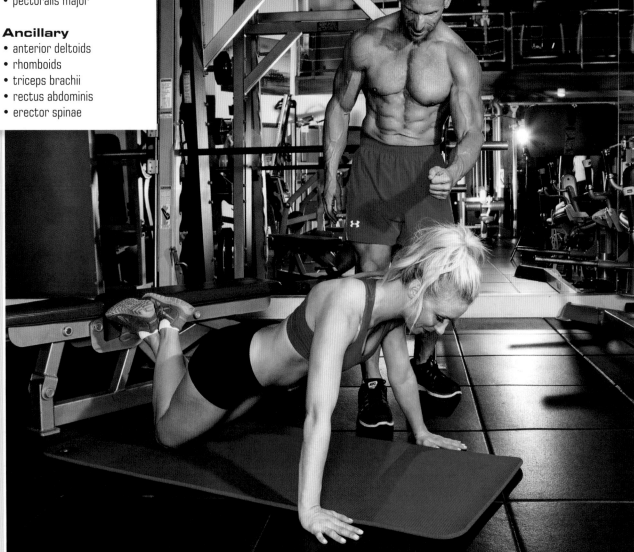

PROPER FORM
Do it right
- Perform slow and controlled repetitions.
- Keep your upper body straight and stabilize your torso throughout.
- Lower yourself until your upper arms are parallel to the ground.

Avoid
- Excessive speed.
- Shallow or bouncy repetitions.
- Allowing your lower back to dip too far.

MODIFICATIONS
Beginner
- A wider hand spacing will decrease the range of motion.

Advanced
- Perform a trational push-up with your legs straight.

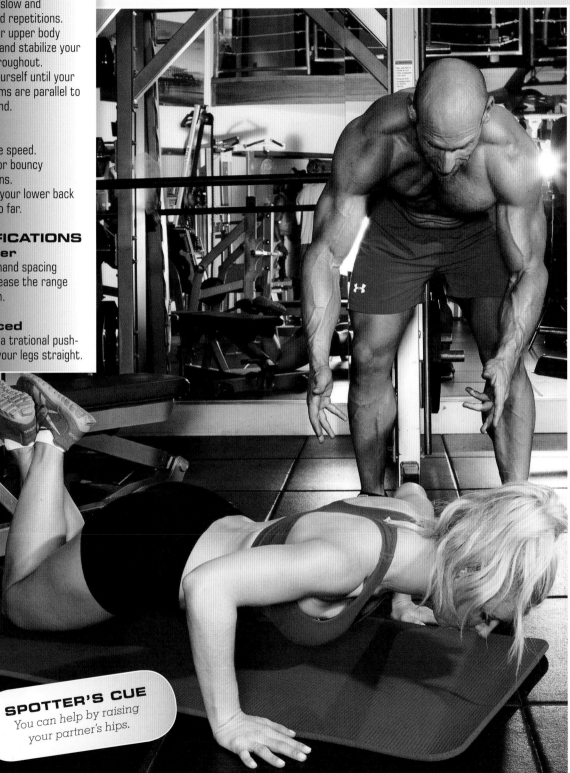

SPOTTER'S CUE
You can help by raising your partner's hips.

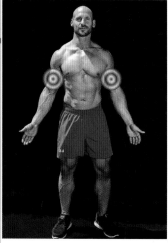

REVERSE BARBELL CURL

1 Stand tall, holding a barbell with an overhand grip approximately shoulder-width apart with your arms fully extended downward.

2 Bend at the elbows as you curl the weight up toward your shoulders in an arced pathway.

3 Lower and repeat for 10 to 12 repetitions.

MUSCLE ACTION
Primary
- biceps brachii

Ancillary
- forearm extensors
- forearm flexors
- rectus abdominis
- erector spinae

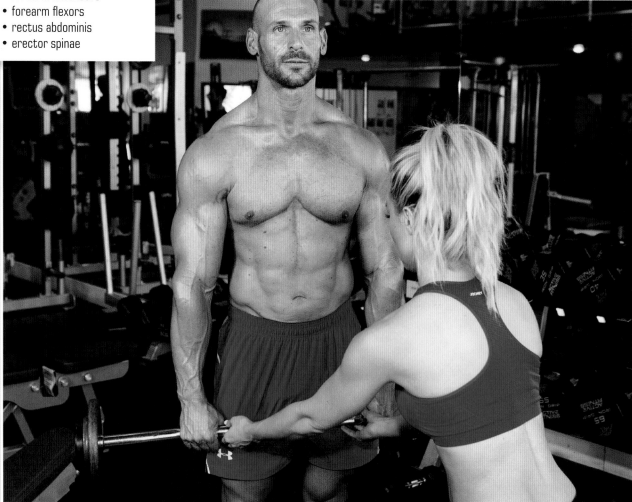

PROPER FORM
Do it right
- Move through a full and controlled range of motion.
- Keep your elbows close to your body.
- Lower the bar slowly.

Avoid
- Using momentum to swing the weight up.
- Flaring your elbows out.
- Excessively using your lower back to complete the movement.

MODIFICATIONS
Beginner
- A wider grip will decrease the range of motion.

Advanced
- Use dumbbells.

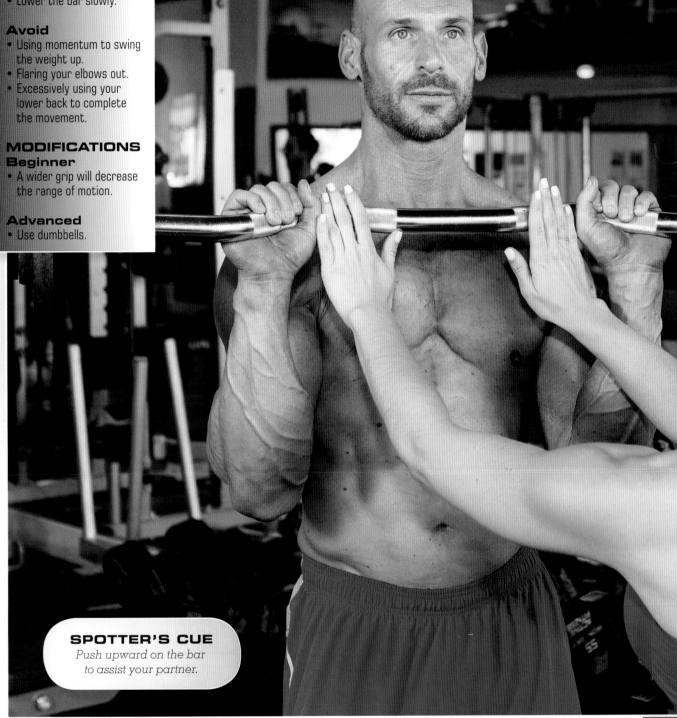

SPOTTER'S CUE
Push upward on the bar to assist your partner.

CABLE CURL

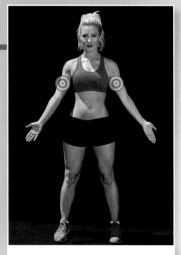

1 Stand tall, holding a bar attachment from a low pulley with an underhand grip approximately shoulder-width apart with your arms fully extended downward.

2 Bend at the elbows as you curl the weight up toward your shoulders in an arced pathway.

3 Lower, and repeat for 12 to 15 repetitions.

MUSCLE ACTION
Primary
• biceps brachii

Ancillary
• forearm extensors
• forearm flexors
• rectus abdominis
• erector spinae

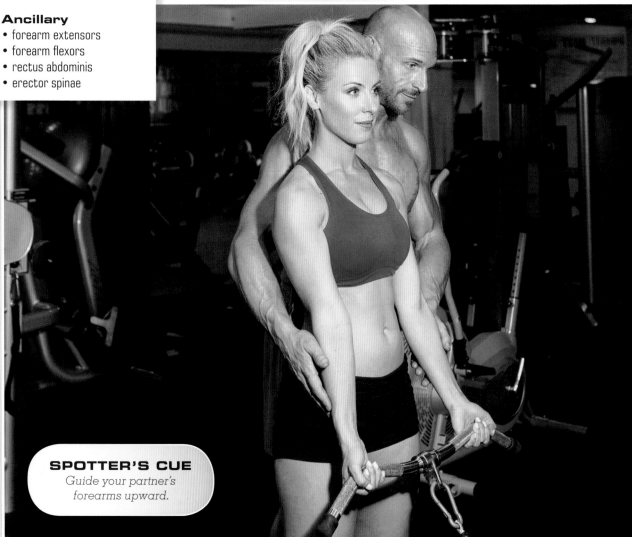

SPOTTER'S CUE
Guide your partner's forearms upward.

PROPER FORM
Do it right
- Move through a full and controlled range of motion.
- Keep your elbows close to your body.
- Lower the bar slowly.

Avoid
- Using momentum to swing the weight up.
- Employing too narrow a grip.
- Excessively using your lower back to complete the movement.

MODIFICATIONS
Beginner
- A wider grip will decrease the range of motion.

Advanced
- Use dumbbells.

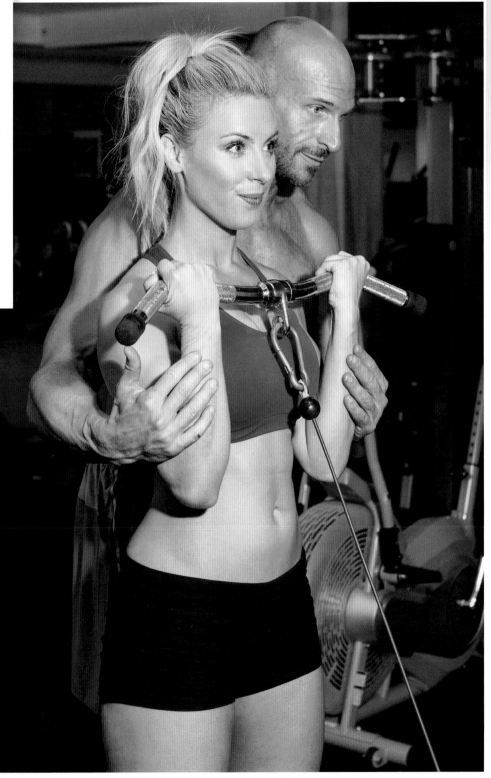

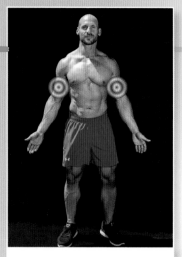

OVERHEAD PULLEY CURL

1 Stand in the middle of a pulley station holding a handle in each hand attached to a high pulley with your arms extended directly out to your sides and slightly above parallel to the ground.

2 Bend the elbows as you curl the weight toward your shoulders.

3 Return to the start position, and repeat for 12 to 15 repetitions.

MUSCLE ACTION
Primary
• biceps brachii

Ancillary
• forearm extensors
• forearm flexors
• rectus abdominis
• erector spinae

SPOTTER'S CUE
Push in at the elbows or forearms.

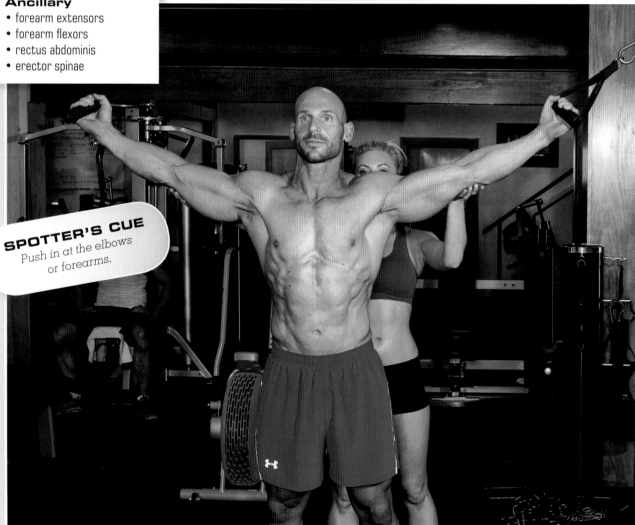

PROPER FORM
Do it right
- Move through a full and controlled range of motion.
- Keep your arms and shoulders elevated.
- Squeeze your biceps at the top of the movement.

Avoid
- Using momentum to swing the weight up.
- Allowing your arms and shoulders to dip.
- An incomplete range of motion.

MODIFICATIONS
Beginner
- Use one arm at a time.

Advanced
- Use dumbbells.

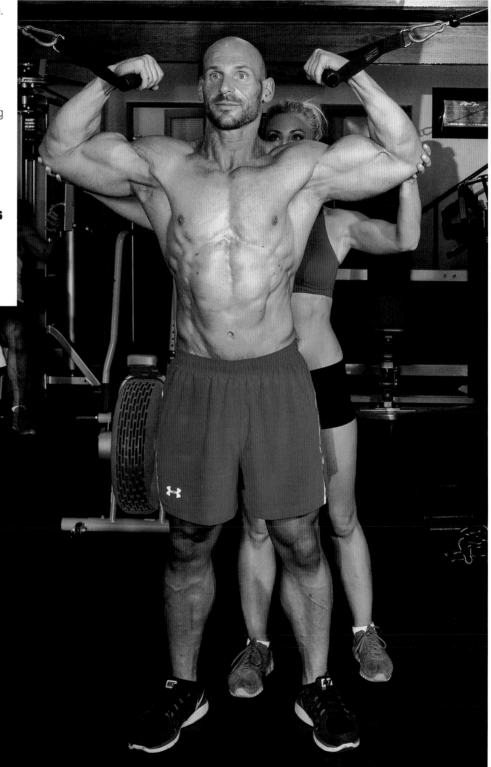

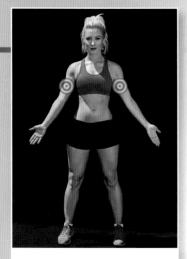

MUSCLE ACTION
Primary
- biceps brachii

Ancillary
- forearm extensors
- forearm flexors

TARGET: BICEPS

CONCENTRATION CURL

1 Sit in the middle of a flat bench with your feet planted wide. Grasp a dumbbell in one hand as you extend your arm downward between your legs, bracing your upper arm against your inner thigh. Rotate the palm of your hand until it is facing forward away from your thigh. Place your other hand on your opposite leg for support.

2 Bend the working elbow, and curl your arm upward in an arced pathway until the weight nearly touches your shoulder.

3 Lower, and repeat for 12 to 15 repetitions per arm.

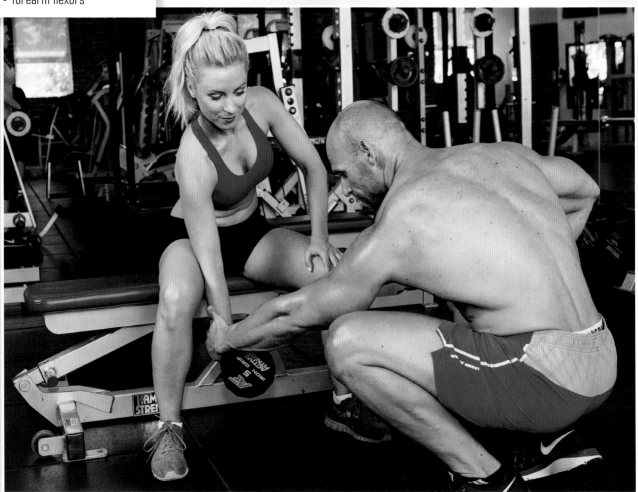

PROPER FORM
Do it right
- Move through a full and controlled range of motion.
- Fully extend your arm at the start of the movement.
- Move slowly.

Avoid
- Using momentum to swing the dumbbell upward.
- Shifting your upper arm away from your thigh.
- Excessively using your shoulder muscles to complete the movement.

MODIFICATIONS
Beginner
- Use a lighter weight.

Advanced
- Use a heavier weight.

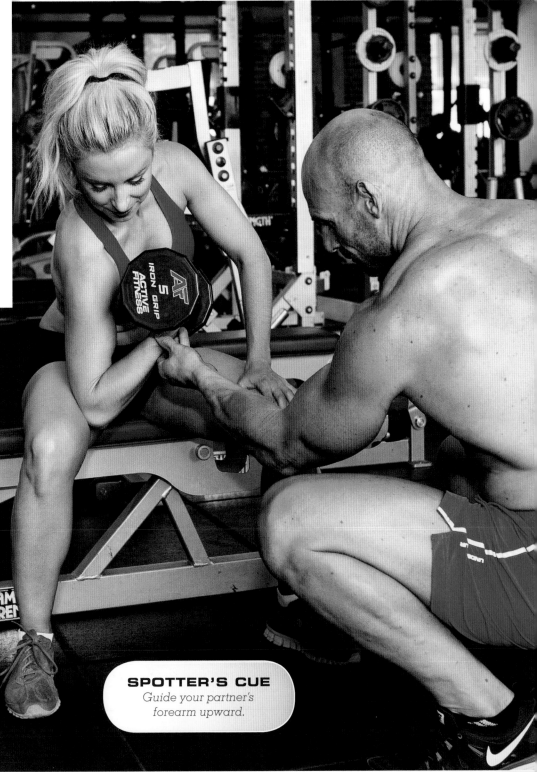

SPOTTER'S CUE
Guide your partner's forearm upward.

SWISS BALL WALL SQUAT

1 Lean against a wall with a Swiss ball positioned at your lower back. Bring your feet slightly forward in a shoulder-width stance with your toes pointing forward and your hands on your hips.

2 While keeping an erect posture, bend your knees, lowering your body until your thighs are parallel to the ground.

3 Push through your heels to return to the starting position. Repeat for 12 to 15 repetitions.

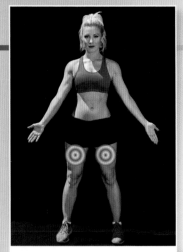

MUSCLE ACTION
Primary
- rectus femoris
- vastus lateralis
- vastus intermedius
- vastus medialis
- gluteus maximus
- biceps femoris
- semitendinosus
- semimembranosus

Ancillary
- erector spinae
- rectus abdominis
- adductor magnus
- soleus
- gastrocnemius

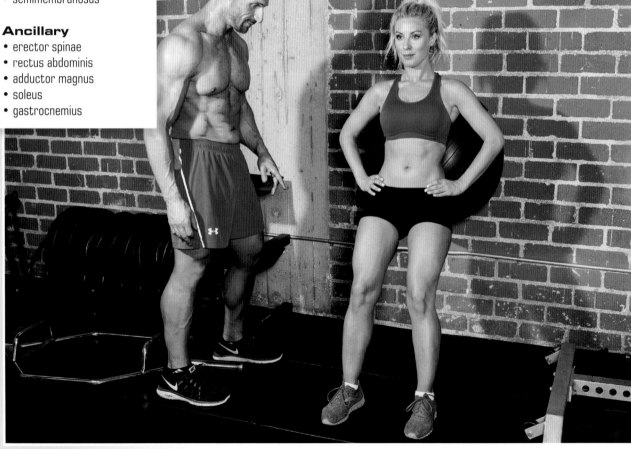

PROPER FORM
Do it right
- Squat until your thighs are parallel to the ground.
- Move through a full and controlled range of motion.
- Push through your heels to drive the movement.

Avoid
- Hyperextending your toes past your feet.
- Descending or dropping too rapidly.
- Pushing through your toes to drive the movement.

MODIFICATIONS
Beginner
- A wider stance will decrease the range of motion.

Advanced
- Keep one foot firmly planted on the ground while raising the other.

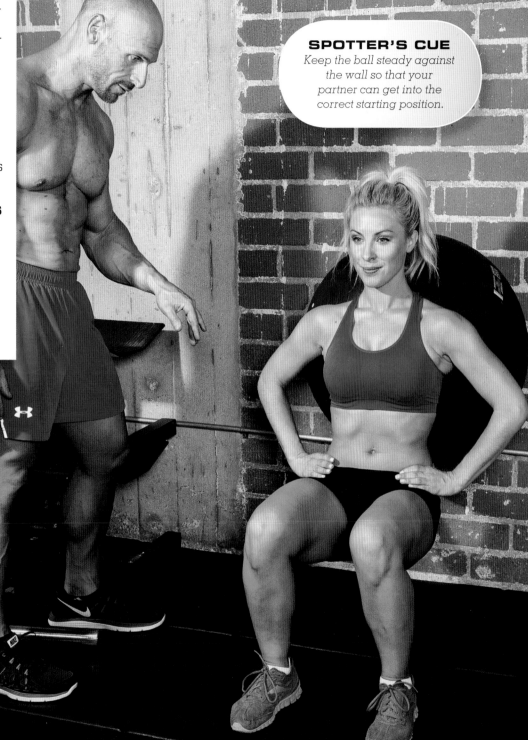

SPOTTER'S CUE
Keep the ball steady against the wall so that your partner can get into the correct starting position.

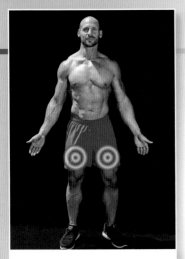

FRONT SQUAT

1 Stand your feet shoulder-width apart in a squat rack with a barbell placed at the upper end. Duck under the bar, and with your shoulders firmly under the bar, cross your arms, lightly resting your hands on the top of the bar.

2 Walk back a step or two, maintaining your shoulder-width stance with your toes straight-on and your knees soft or slightly bent.

3 Bend your knees, lowering yourself until your thighs are parallel to the ground while keeping an erect posture.

4 Push through your heels to return to the starting position. Repeat for 12 to 15 repetitions.

MUSCLE ACTION
Primary
- rectus femoris
- vastus lateralis
- vastus intermedius
- vastus medialis
- gluteus maximus
- biceps femoris
- semitendinosus
- semimembranosus

Ancillary
- erector spinae
- rectus abdominis
- adductor magnus
- soleus
- gastrocnemius

SPOTTER'S CUE
Get behind your partner and lift from under the armpits.

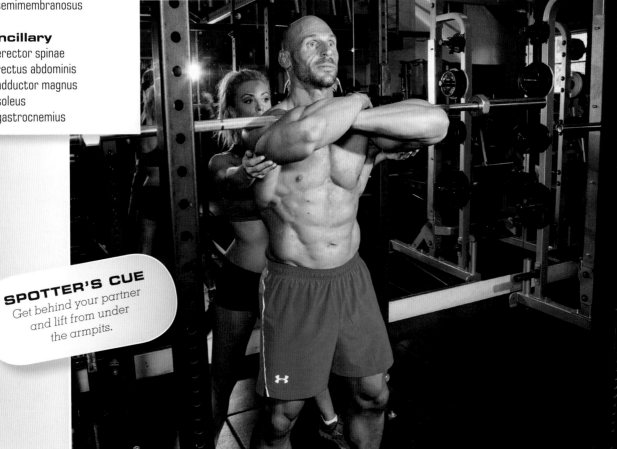

PROPER FORM
Do it right
- Squat until your thighs are parallel to the ground.
- Keep the bar firmly in place across your shoulders.
- Push through your heels to drive the movement.

Avoid
- Hyperextending your toes past your feet.
- Allowing the bar to roll off your shoulders.
- Pushing through your toes to drive the movement.

MODIFICATIONS
Beginner
- A wider stance will decrease the range of motion.

Advanced
- A closer stance will increase the range of motion.

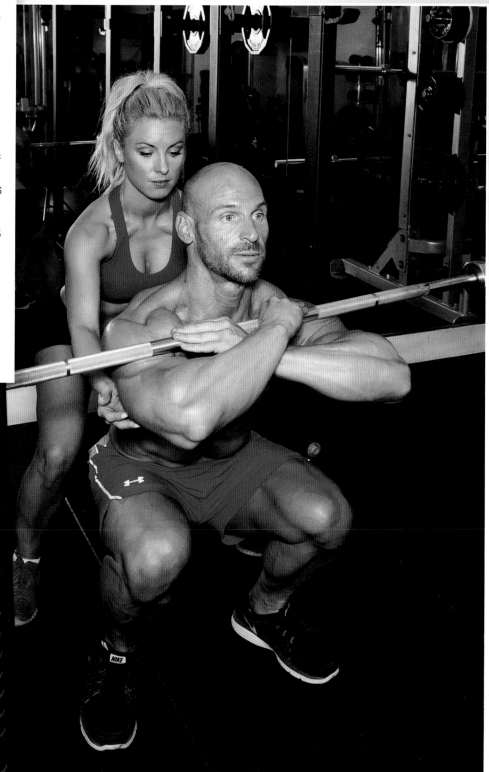

SINGLE-LEG PRESS

1 Position yourself on a leg press machine with one foot on the platform and the other on the floor. Press the platform up to full knee extension, unhook the latches and then lower it toward your chest until your thigh and calf form a 90-degree angle.

2 Extend through your heel to straighten your leg. Repeat for 12 to 15 repetitions per leg.

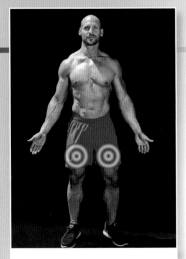

MUSCLE ACTION
Primary
• rectus femoris
• vastus lateralis
• vastus intermedius
• vastus medialis
• gluteus maximus
• biceps femoris
• semitendinosus
• semimembranosus

Ancillary
• rectus abdominis
• soleus
• gastrocnemius

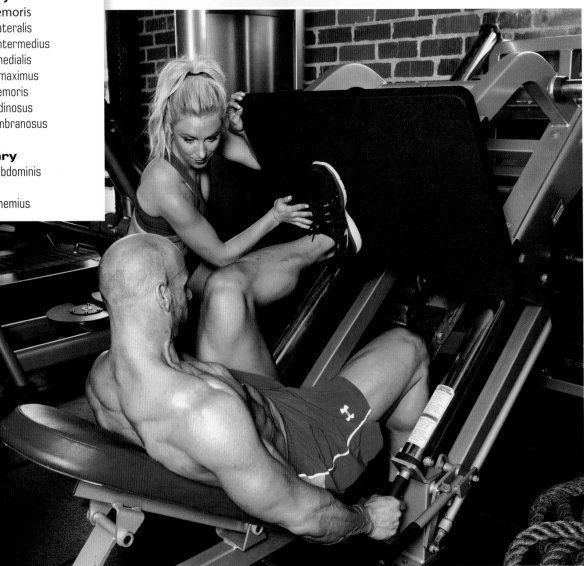

PROPER FORM
Do it right
- Push through your heel to drive the movement.
- Straighten your working leg to just shy of lockout.
- Keep your foot planted more to the side than the center.

Avoid
- Leading with your toes to drive the movement.
- Lowering too far into your rib cage.
- Allowing your pelvis to rise from the seat.

MODIFICATIONS
Beginner
- Use both legs.

Advanced
- Use a heavier resistance.

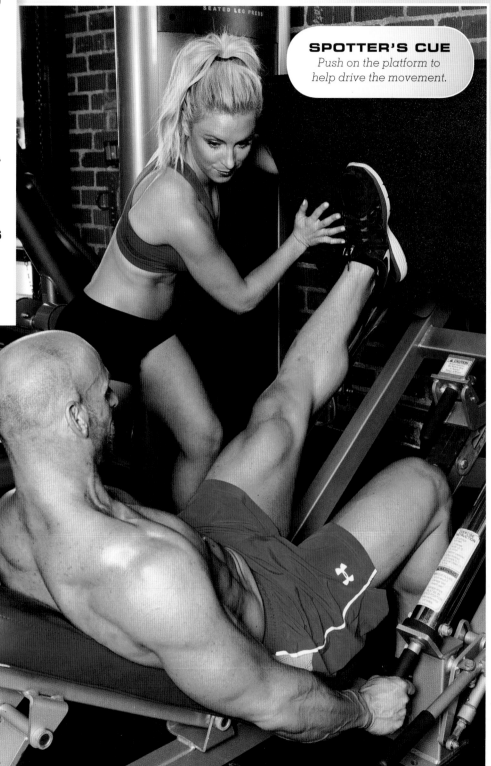

SPOTTER'S CUE
Push on the platform to help drive the movement.

BENCH LUNGE

1 Stand in front of a flat bench with one leg placed ahead on the ground and the opposite back of the foot placed on the bench.

2 Place your hand on your hip and maintain an erect posture while bending both legs until your front thigh is parallel to the ground.

3 Push through the front heel to raise yourself to full extension, and repeat for 12 to 15 repetitions per leg.

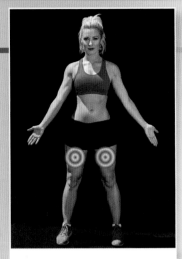

MUSCLE ACTION
Primary
- rectus femoris
- vastus lateralis
- vastus intermedius
- vastus medialis
- gluteus maximus
- biceps femoris
- semitendinosus
- semimembranosus

Ancillary
- erector spinae
- rectus abdominis
- adductor magnus
- soleus
- gastrocnemius

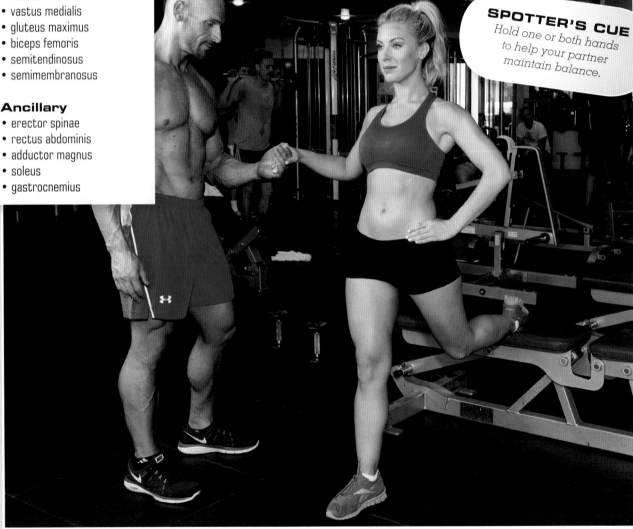

SPOTTER'S CUE
Hold one or both hands to help your partner maintain balance.

PROPER FORM
Do it right
- Push through your front heel to drive the movement.
- Lunge downward until your front thigh is parallel to the ground.
- Keep your eyes focused on a spot ahead of you to keep balanced.

Avoid
- Allowing your knee to hyperextend past your foot.
- Allowing your back foot to wobble or shift.
- Slouching.

MODIFICATIONS
Beginner
- Hold a pole planted on the ground for support.

Advanced
- Hold a pair of dumbbells.

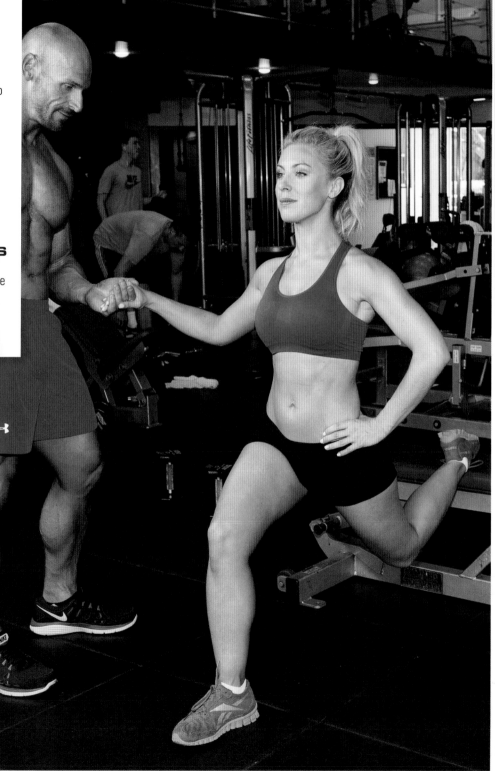

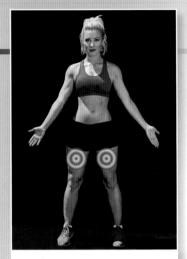

SINGLE-LEG EXTENSION

1 Sit at a leg extension machine with both feet under the roller pad and grip the hand rests at your sides. The roller pad should be against the lower part of your shin, but not in contact with the ankle. Adjust the seat so that the pivot point is in line with your knee.

2 Extend one leg up to full extension.

3 Lower and repeat for 12 to 15 repetitions per leg.

MUSCLE ACTION
Primary
- rectus femoris
- vastus lateralis
- vastus intermedius
- vastus medialis

Ancillary
- rectus abdominis
- tibialis anterior

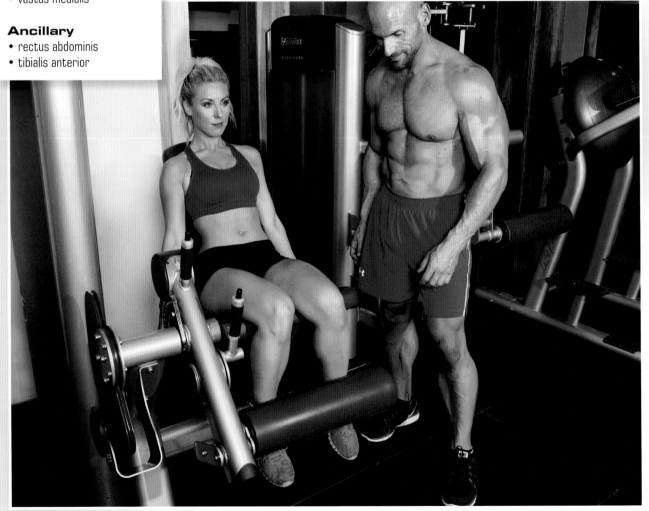

PROPER FORM
Do it right
- Move through a controlled downward range of motion.
- Perform an explosive but controlled positive (raising).
- A peak contraction at the top of the movement.

Avoid
- Speedy or bouncy repetitions.
- Allowing momentum to drive the movement.
- Leaning too far forward to cheat the weight up.

MODIFICATIONS
Beginner
- Use both legs.

Advanced
- Use a heavier resistance.

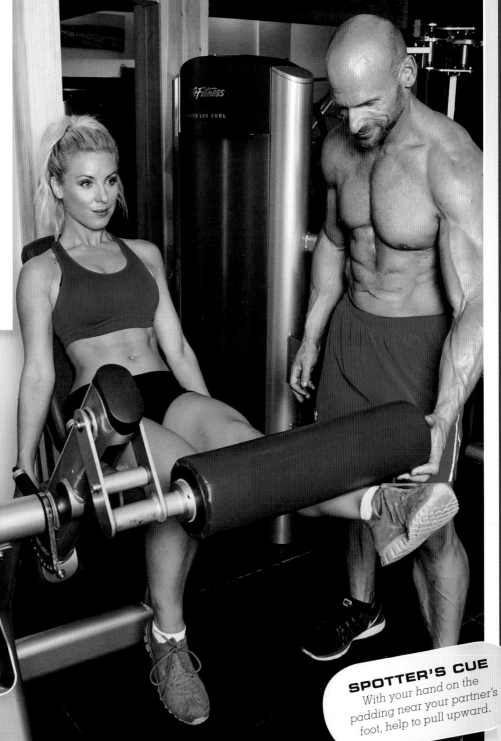

SPOTTER'S CUE
With your hand on the padding near your partner's foot, help to pull upward.

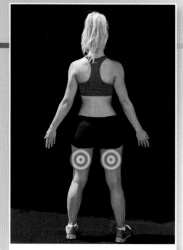

DUMBBELL STIFF-LEGGED DEADLIFT

1 Hold a pair of dumbbells in front of you with your palms facing your thighs, and, keeping a flat back, lean forward at the waist. Maintain soft or slightly bent knees as you stretch your arms toward the ground.

2 Slowly rise until the weights are just above your knees, and then squeeze your glutes at the top. Repeat for 12 to 15 repetitions.

MUSCLE ACTION
Primary
- biceps femoris
- semitendinosus
- semimembranosus
- gluteus maximus

Ancillary
- gastrocnemius
- erector spinae

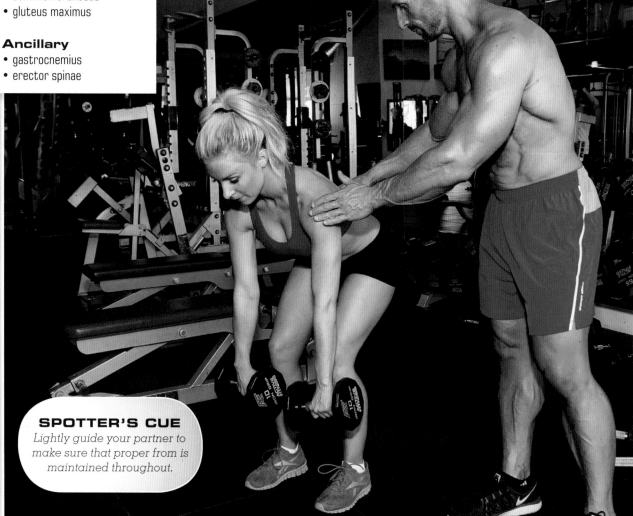

SPOTTER'S CUE

Lightly guide your partner to make sure that proper from is maintained throughout.

PROPER FORM
Do it right
- Move through a full and controlled range of motion.
- Maintain a flat back throughout.
- Achieve a full stretch at the beginning of the movement.

Avoid
- Speedy repetitions.
- Completely standing up.
- Rounding your back.

MODIFICATIONS
Beginner
- Use a barbell.

Advanced
- Stand on one leg.

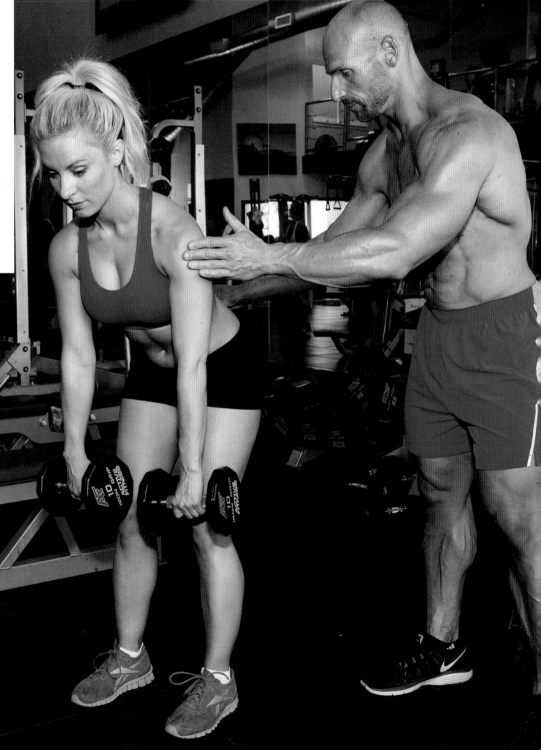

KETTLEBELL STIFF-LEGGED DEADLIFT

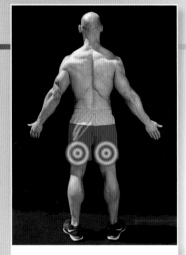

1 Hold a kettlebell in front of you with your palms facing your thighs, and, keeping a flat back, lean forward at the waist. Maintain soft or slightly bent knees as you stretch your arms toward the ground.

2 Slowly rise to full lockout, and then squeeze your glutes at the top. Repeat for 12 to 15 repetitions.

MUSCLE ACTION
Primary
- biceps femoris
- semitendinosus
- semimembranosus
- gluteus maximus

Ancillary
- gastrocnemius
- erector spinae

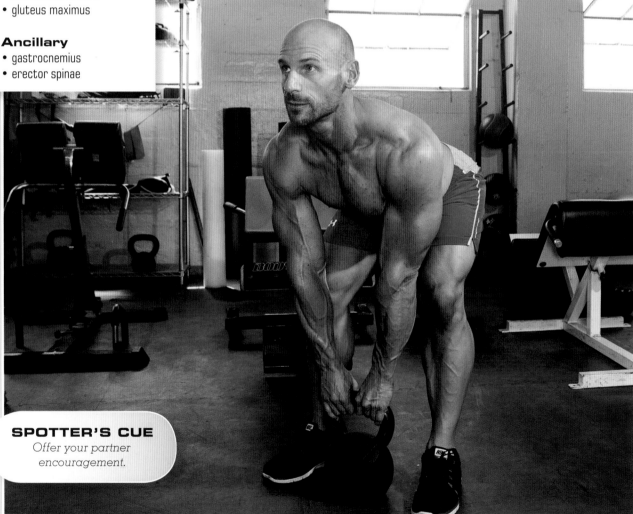

SPOTTER'S CUE
Offer your partner encouragement.

PROPER FORM
Do it right
- Move through a full and controlled range of motion.
- Maintain a flat back throughout.
- Achieve a full stretch at the beginning of the movement.

Avoid
- Speedy repetitions.
- Leaning too far forward.
- Rounding your back.

MODIFICATIONS
Beginner
- Use a pair of dumbbells.

Advanced
- Stand on one leg.

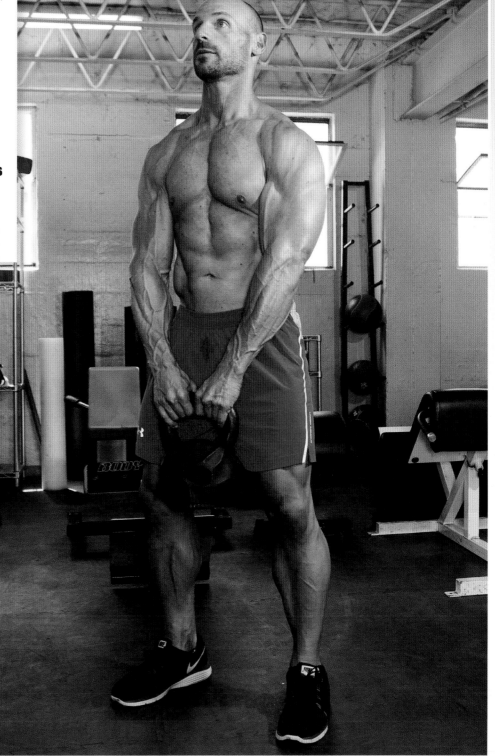

SWISS BALL RAISE

1 Lie on your back with your arms at your sides in front of a Swiss ball. Bend your knees, and place your feet flat on the ball.

2 Push through your heels as you simultaneously raise your lower body off the ground, squeezing your glutes at the top.

3 Lower, return to the downward position, and then repeat for 12 to 15 repetitions.

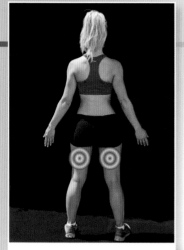

MUSCLE ACTION
Primary
- biceps femoris
- semitendinosus
- semimembranosus
- gluteus maximus

Ancillary
- gastrocnemius
- rectus abdominis
- erector spinae

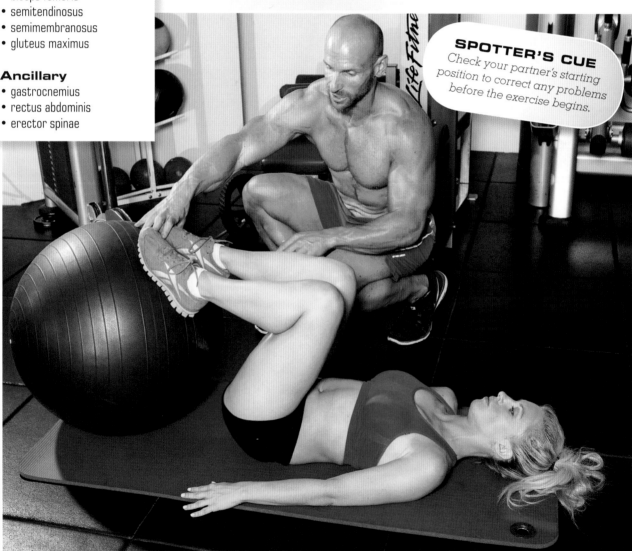

SPOTTER'S CUE
Check your partner's starting position to correct any problems before the exercise begins.

PROPER FORM
Do it right
- Keep your hips elevated.
- Keep your heels firmly grounded on the ball.
- Stabilize your torso.

Avoid
- Straightening your legs.
- Speedy repetitions.
- Rotating your torso.

MODIFICATIONS
Beginner
- Perform fewer repetitions.

Advanced
- Try it with one leg.

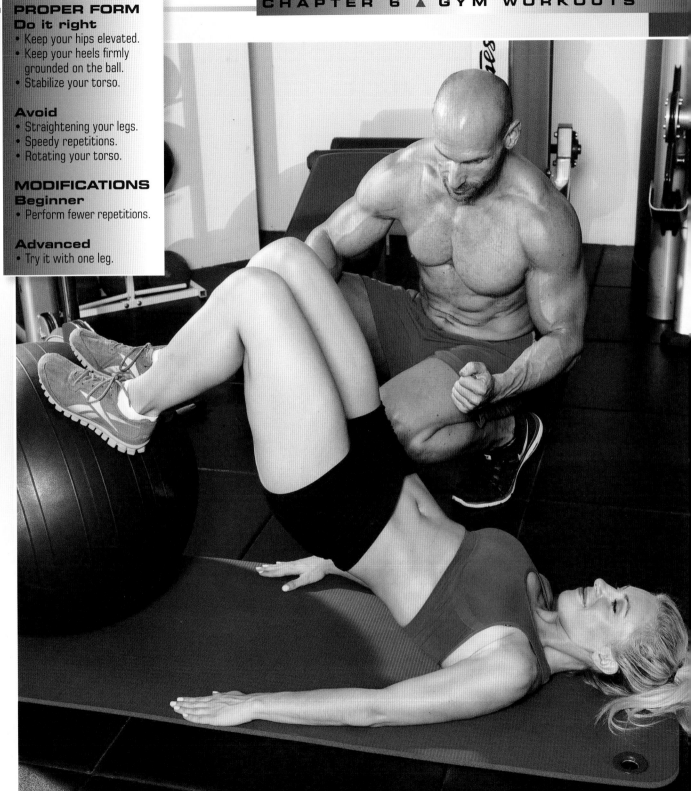

ONE-LEGGED SWISS BALL CURL

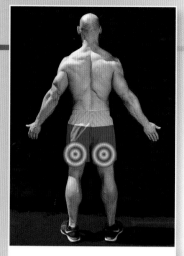

1 Lie on your back in front of a Swiss ball with your arms at your sides. Place your heel on the ball, and then raise one leg straight up. Using your heel like a claw to hold the ball into place, raise your lower body off the ground while keeping it in one straight line.

2 Bend the working leg, and bring the ball in toward your glutes while keeping your body elevated off the ground.

3 Return to the starting position. Repeat for 12 to 15 repetitions per leg.

MUSCLE ACTION
Primary
- biceps femoris
- semitendinosus
- semimembranosus
- gluteus maximus

Ancillary
- gastrocnemius
- rectus abdominis
- erector spinae

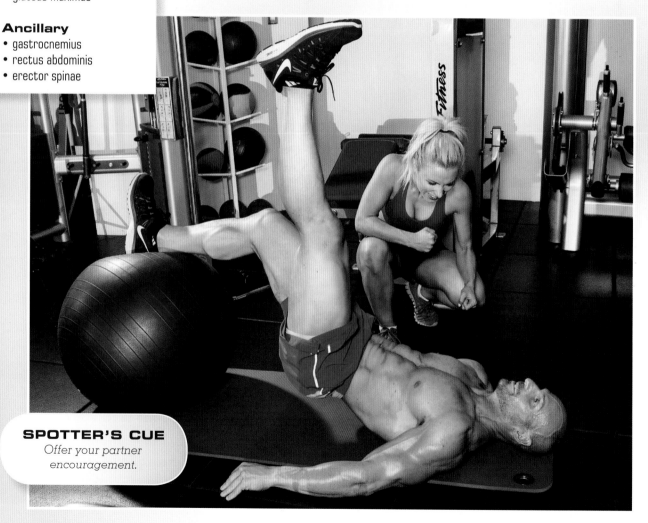

SPOTTER'S CUE
Offer your partner encouragement.

PROPER FORM
Do it right
- Keep your leg bent throughout.
- Keep your heel firmly grounded on the ball.
- Keep your torso elevated.

Avoid
- Allowing your hips to dip.
- Speedy repetitions.
- Rotating your torso.

MODIFICATIONS
Beginner
- Perform fewer reps.

Advanced
- Wear an ankle weight.

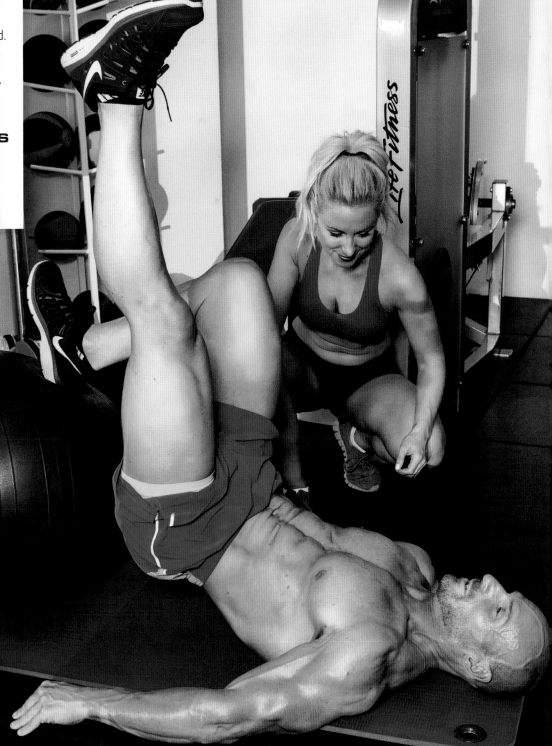

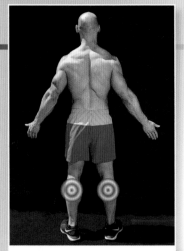

SEATED CALF RAISE

1 Sit at a calf machine with your thighs under the pad and the tips of your toes on the platform.

2 Rise up on your toes as you release the weight mechanism, and place your hands on the rests.

3 Lower your heels, and then rise up on your toes, flexing your calf muscles at the topmost position. Repeat for 12 to 15 repetitions.

MUSCLE ACTION
Primary
- gastrocnemius
- soleus

Ancillary
- tibialis anterior

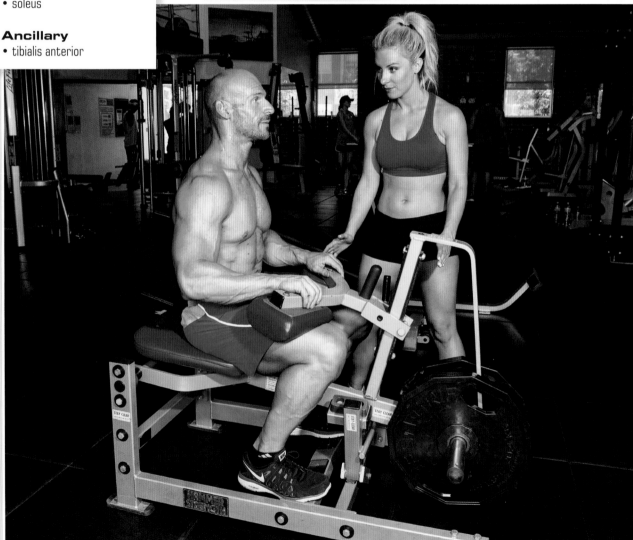

PROPER FORM
Do it right
- Move through a full and controlled range of motion.
- Keep your toes pointed forward.
- Contract your calf muscles at the top of the movement.

Avoid
- Partial repetitions.
- Bouncy or speedy repetitions.
- Having too much of your feet on the platform.

MODIFICATIONS
Beginner
- Use less resistance.

Advanced
- Use one foot at a time.

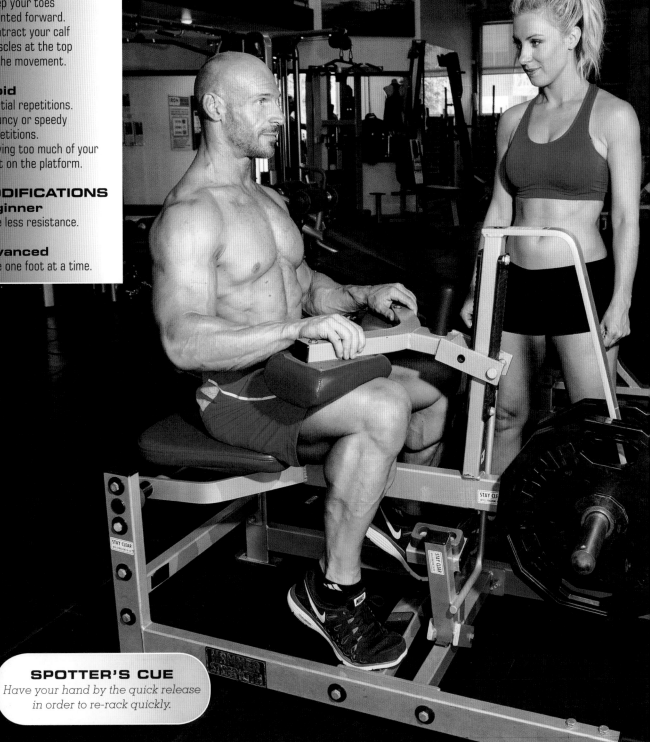

SPOTTER'S CUE
Have your hand by the quick release in order to re-rack quickly.

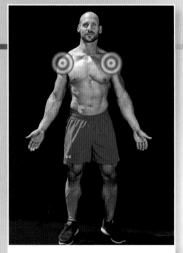

SMITH MACHINE SHOULDER PRESS

1 Place a flat bench underneath a Smith machine, and sit with an overhand grip on the bar, your hands slightly wider than shoulder width.

2 Lift and twist the bar to free the weight, and lower it to just below your chin.

3 Push overhead to full lockout, and then repeat for 8 to 12 repetitions.

MUSCLE ACTION
Primary
- anterior deltoids

ANCILLARY
- medial deltoids
- triceps brachii
- trapezius
- rhomboids
- rectus abdominis
- erector spinae

SPOTTER'S CUE
Push at the elbows to offer assistance.

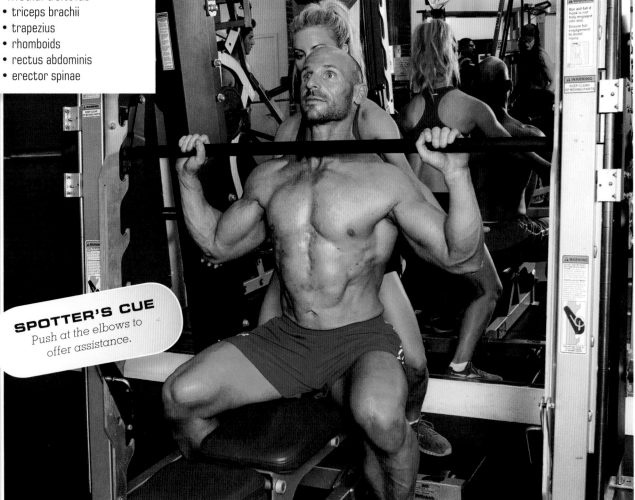

PROPER FORM
Do it right
- Perform slow and controlled repetitions.
- Use a bench with a back for greater stability and support.
- Keep the bar in front of your shoulders.

Avoid
- Pressing the weight behind your neck.
- An incomplete range of motion.
- Arching your back.

MODIFICATIONS
Beginner
- Use a lighter weight.

Advanced
- Use a close underhand grip or dumbbells.

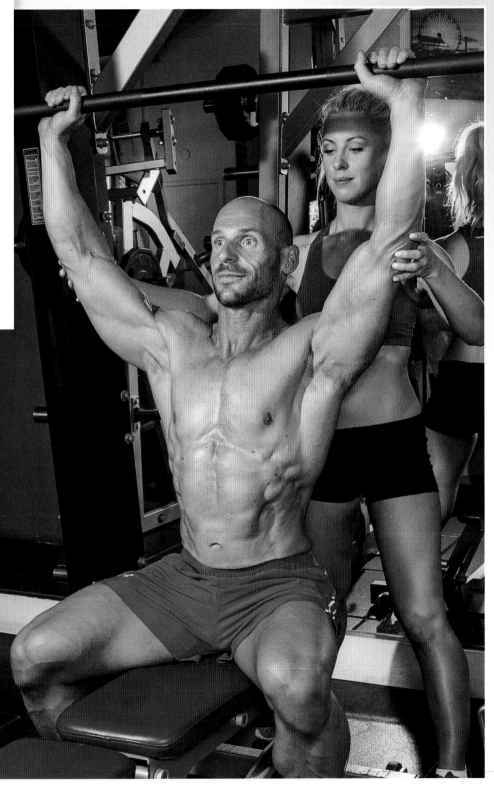

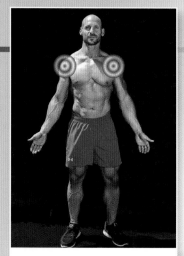

KETTLEBELL ONE-ARM CLEAN AND PRESS

1 Stand while holding a kettlebell in one hand.

2 Flip the kettlebell up until it is nearly touching your shoulder.

3 Rotate your palm as you push overhead.

4 Reverse, and return to the starting position. Repeat for 8 to 12 repetitions per arm.

MUSCLE ACTION

Primary
- anterior deltoids
- medial deltoids
- posterior deltoids
- triceps brachii
- trapezius

Ancillary
- rectus abdominis
- erector spinae
- rhomboids
- gastrocnemius
- soleus

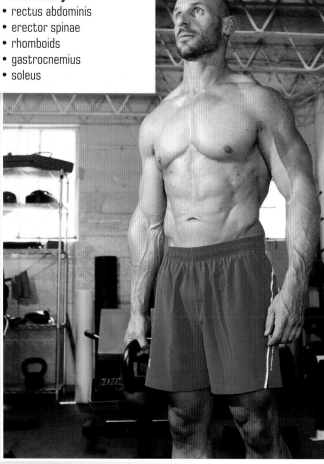

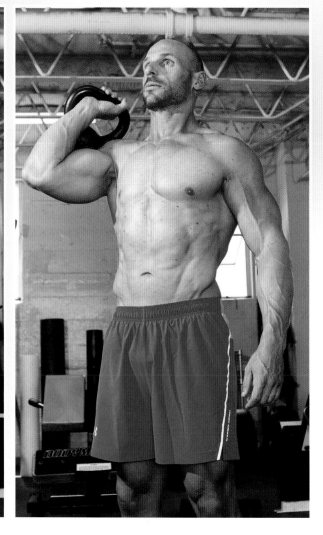

PROPER FORM
Do it right
- Keep your body stabilized.
- Keep the kettlebell close to your body.
- Move through a full and controlled range of motion.

Avoid
- Overarching your back.
- Placing too much stress on your wrists.
- Excessive speed or momentum.

MODIFICATIONS
Beginner
- Use a lighter weight.

Advanced
- Try it with a kettlebell in each hand.

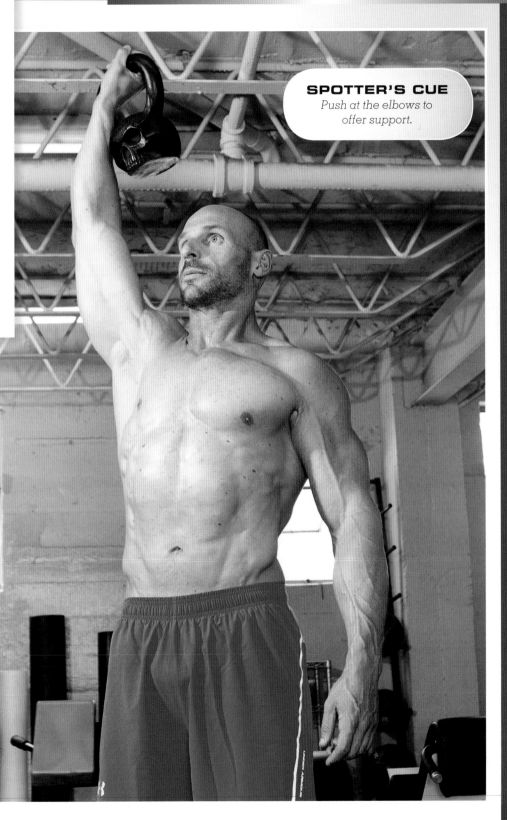

SPOTTER'S CUE
Push at the elbows to offer support.

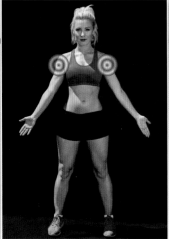

PRONE SHOULDER PRESS

1 Lie facedown on an incline bench with your legs bent and supported on the lower pad and your torso straight. Grasp a light dumbbell in each hand with palms down directly in front of your shoulders.

2 Extend your arms straight in front of you and arcing in at the extended position.

3 Return to the starting position along the same pathway. Repeat for 10 to 12 repetitions.

MUSCLE ACTION
Primary
- anterior deltoids
- medial deltoids
- posterior deltoids

Ancillary
- trapezius
- rhomboids
- latissimus dorsi
- erector spinae

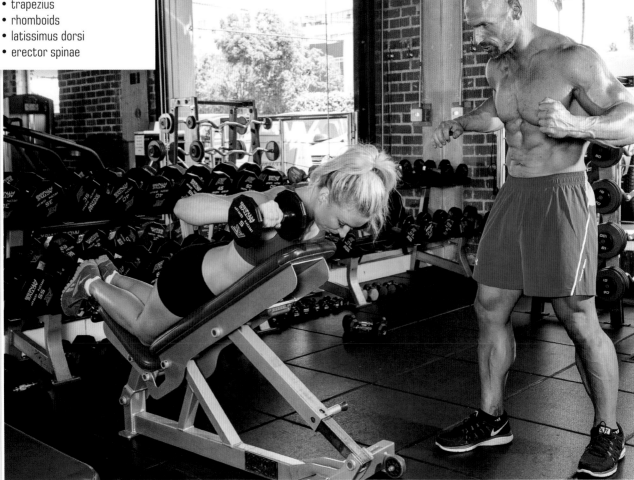

PROPER FORM
Do it right
- Maintain an elongated torso throughout.
- Keep your hands at shoulder level.
- Keep your head down to avoid neck strain.

Avoid
- Allowing your arms to drop.
- Excessive speed or momentum.
- Allowing your chest to rise off the bench.

MODIFICATIONS
Beginner
- Use a lighter weight.

Advanced
- Alternate arms.

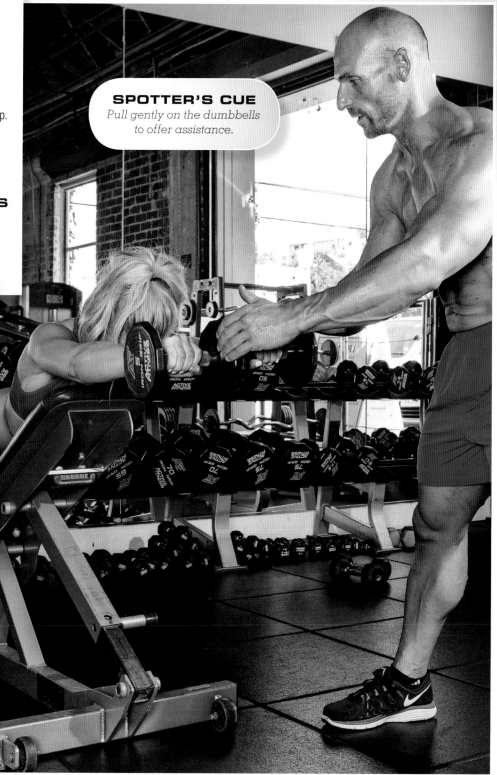

SPOTTER'S CUE
Pull gently on the dumbbells to offer assistance.

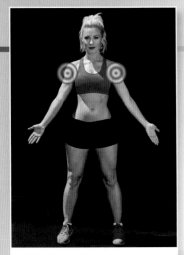

ALTERNATING FRONT DUMBBELL RAISE

1 Sit up tall grasping a pair of dumbbells at your sides with your palms facing each other.

2 Maintaining a very slight bend at the elbow, raise one arm straight up until it is parallel to the ground, rotating your wrist so that your palm faces downward at the topmost portion of the repetition.

3 Follow downward along the same pathway, and then perform on the other arm for 10 to 12 repetitions per arm.

MUSCLE ACTION
Primary
- anterior deltoids

Ancillary
- trapezius
- rhomboids
- forearm extensors
- forearm flexors

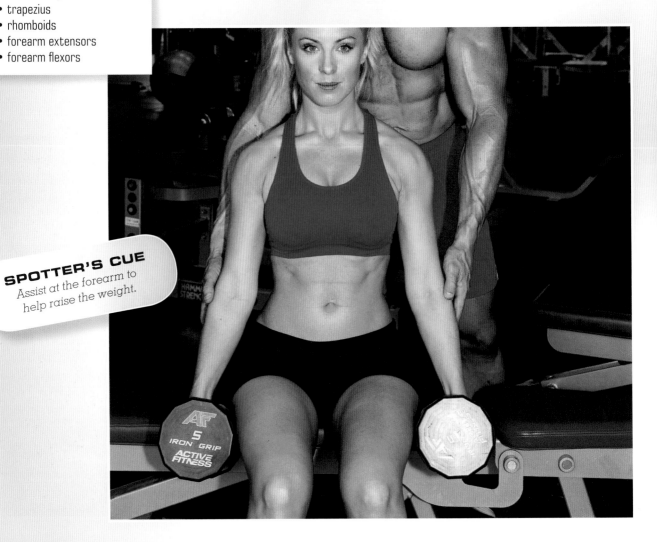

SPOTTER'S CUE
Assist at the forearm to help raise the weight.

PROPER FORM
Do it right
- Maintain an erect posture throughout.
- Keep your working arm slightly bent.
- Raise your working arm parallel to the ground.

Avoid
- Arcing out before raising upward.
- Keeping your arm completely straight.
- Excessive speed or momentum.

MODIFICATIONS
Beginner
- Use a lighter weight.

Advanced
- Perform with both arms simultaneously.

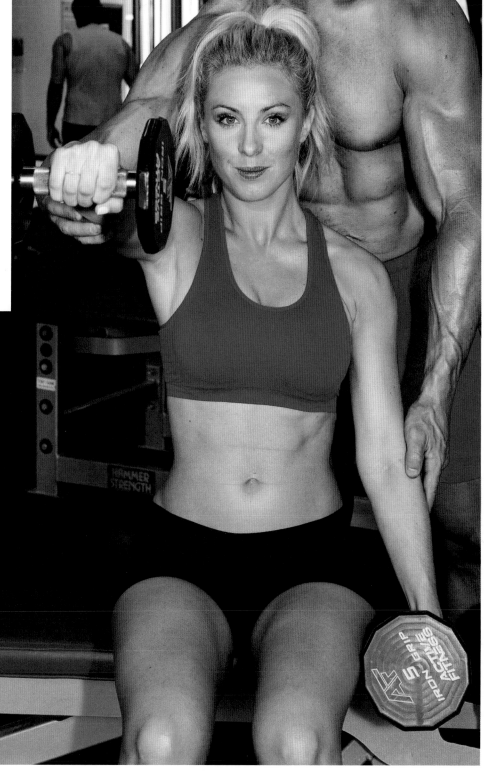

CABLE LATERAL RAISE

1 Stand in a cable station holding one pulley attachment set at the bottom position.

2 Pull your arm directly to the side in an arced path with a slight bend at the elbow until your arm is parallel to the ground.

3 Lower, and repeat for 10 to 12 repetitions per side.

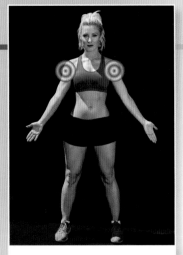

MUSCLE ACTION
Primary
- medial deltoids

Ancillary
- trapezius
- rhomboids
- forearm extensors
- forearm flexors

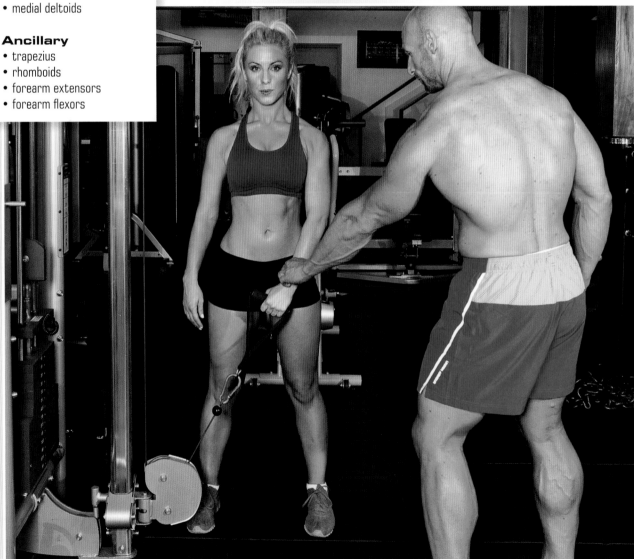

PROPER FORM
Do it right
- Maintain an erect posture.
- Keep your working arm slightly bent.
- Point your thumb slightly downward as you raise your arm.

Avoid
- Raising your arm above parallel to the ground.
- Excessive speed or momentum.
- Allowing your elbow to drop lower than your wrist.

MODIFICATIONS
Beginner
- Use a lighter weight.

Advanced
- Use two handles to perform with both arms simultaneously.

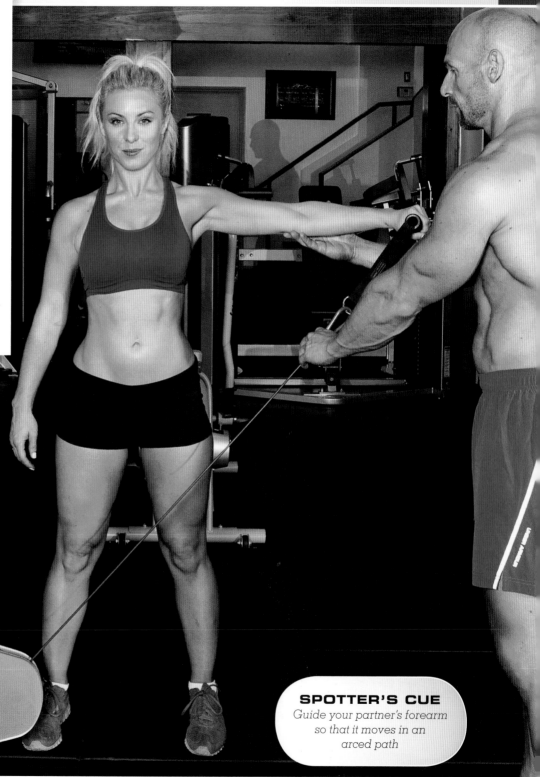

SPOTTER'S CUE
Guide your partner's forearm so that it moves in an arced path

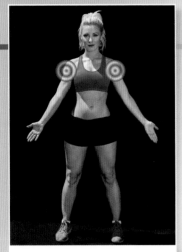

DUMBBELL UPRIGHT ROW

1 Stand while holding a pair of dumbbells in front of your thighs with your palms facing inward.

2 Leading with your elbows, raise your arms, and keep them close to your body.

3 Lower, and repeat for 10 to 12 repetitions.

MUSCLE ACTION
Primary
• medial deltoids

Ancillary
• trapezius
• rhomboids
• forearm extensors
• forearm flexors

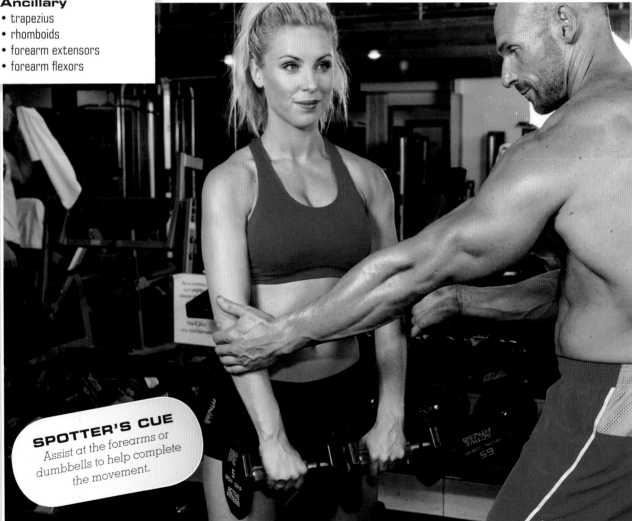

SPOTTER'S CUE
Assist at the forearms or dumbbells to help complete the movement.

PROPER FORM
Do it right
- Keep the dumbbells close to your body.
- Lead with your elbows.
- Raise the dumbbells to chin level.

Avoid
- Dropping your elbows.
- Shifting the dumbbells away from your body.
- Excessive speed or momentum.

MODIFICATIONS
Beginner
- Use a barbell.

Advanced
- Alternate arms.

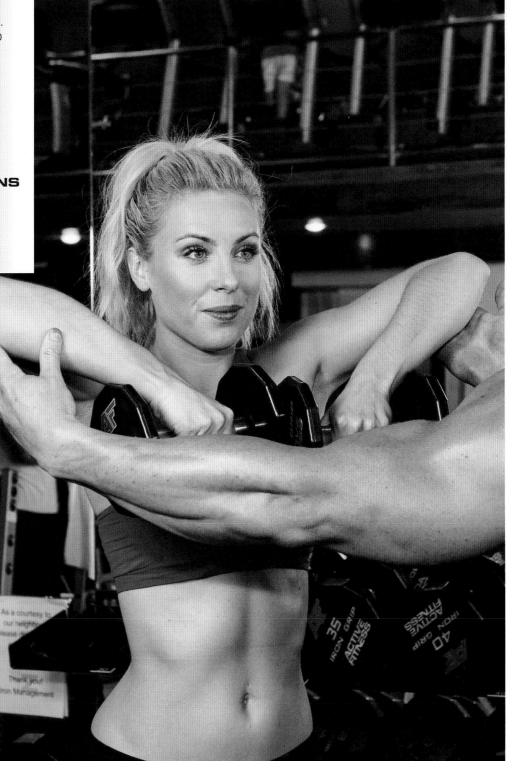

BENCH REAR LATERAL RAISE

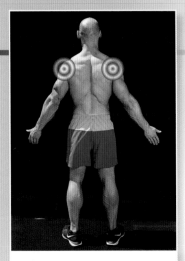

1 Lie facedown on an incline bench with your legs bent and supported on the lower pad and your torso straight. Grasp a dumbbell in each hand aligned directly below your shoulders.

2 Push your arms out to your sides in an arced path with your elbows slightly bent.

3 Return to the starting position along the same pathway. Repeat for 10 to 12 repetitions.

MUSCLE ACTION
Primary
• posterior deltoids

Ancillary
• trapezius
• rhomboids
• forearm extensors
• forearm flexors

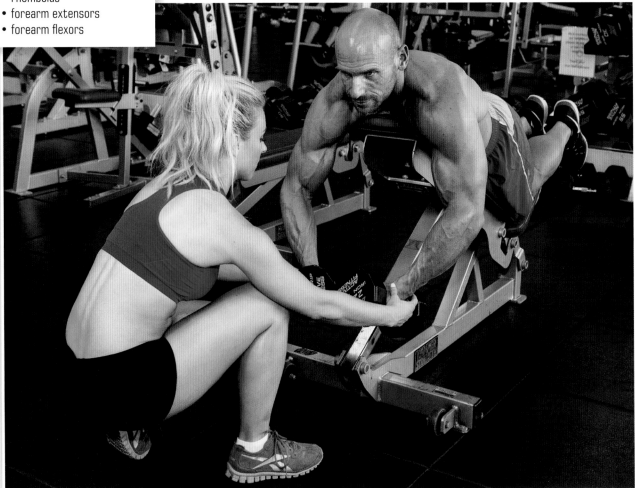

PROPER FORM
Do it right
- Maintain an elongated torso throughout.
- Keep your arms slightly bent.
- Move through an arc-like range of motion.

Avoid
- Excessive speed or momentum.
- Raising your hips.
- Leaning too far back.

MODIFICATIONS
Beginner
- Use a lighter weight.

Advanced
- Alternate arms.

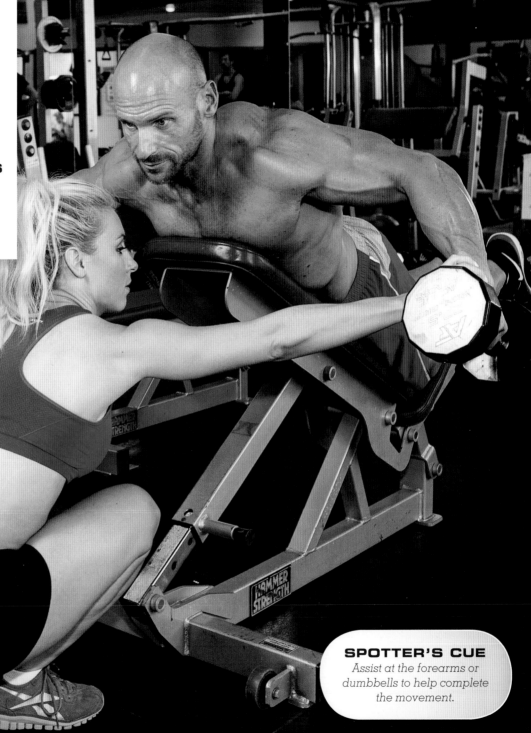

SPOTTER'S CUE
Assist at the forearms or dumbbells to help complete the movement.

LYING DUMBBELL EXTENSION

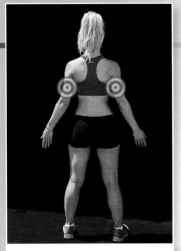

1 Lie back on a flat bench holding a pair of dumbbells with your palms facing each other. While keeping the upper arms braced, bend your elbows, stretching your forearms behind your head.

2 Extend your arms until they are directly above your shoulders. Repeat for 10 to 12 repetitions.

MUSCLE ACTION
Primary
- triceps brachii

Ancillary
- anterior deltoids
- pectoralis major
- rectus abdominis

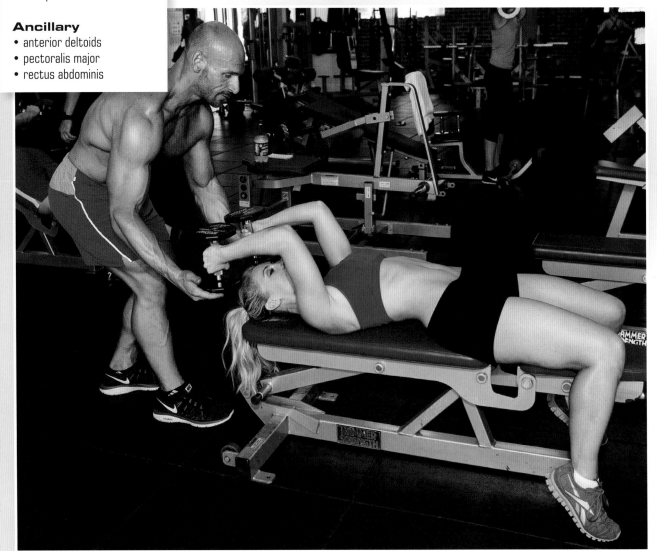

PROPER FORM
Do it right
- Achieve a full stretch behind your head.
- Keep your torso stabilized.
- Keep your elbows in.

Avoid
- Excessive speed.
- Knocking yourself in the head with the weights.
- Flaring your elbows.

MODIFICATIONS
Beginner
- Use a barbell.

Advanced
- Use one arm at a time.

SPOTTER'S CUE

Assist at the forearms or dumbbells to help complete the movement.

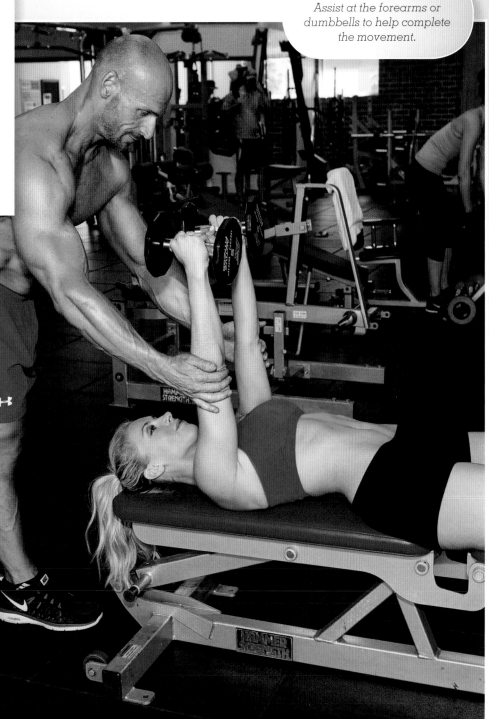

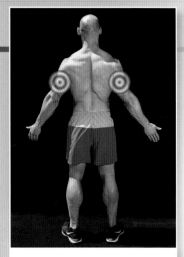

VERTICAL DIP

1 Stand in front of a vertical dip station with your hands on the bars. Lower yourself until your upper arms are parallel to the ground.

2 Push up to full lockout for 10 to 12 repetitions.

MUSCLE ACTION
Primary
- triceps brachii

Ancillary
- anterior deltoids
- pectoralis major
- rhomboids
- rectus abdominis

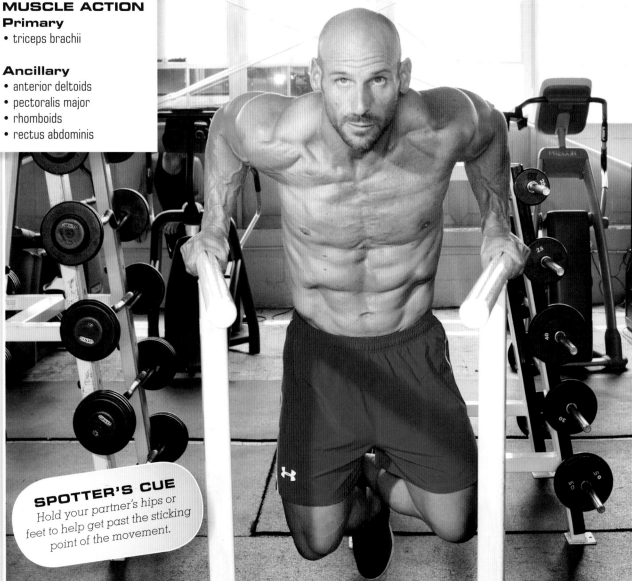

SPOTTER'S CUE
Hold your partner's hips or feet to help get past the sticking point of the movement.

PROPER FORM
Do it right
- Perform controlled repetitions.
- Keep your upper body straight and your torso stabilized.
- Lower yourself until your upper arms are parallel to the ground.

Avoid
- Excessive speed.
- Shallow or bouncy repetitions.
- Leaning too far forward.

MODIFICATIONS
Beginner
- Try the Bench Dip version (see page 150–151).

Advanced
- Drape a heavy chain over your shoulders to add greater resistance.

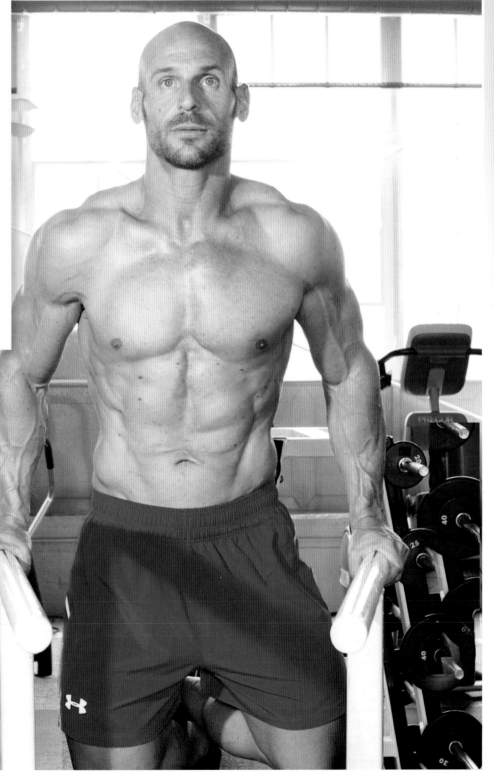

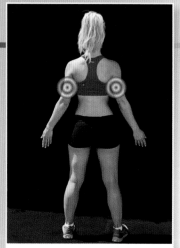

BENCH DIP

1 Place two flat benches side by side. Sit on one on the inner edge of one of them, and grip the edges. Rest your heels on the bench in front of you.

2 Slide your off the bench, and lower your body until your upper arms are parallel to the ground.

3 Push up to full extension, and then repeat for 10 to 12 repetitions.

MUSCLE ACTION
Primary
• triceps brachii

Ancillary
• anterior deltoids
• pectoralis major
• rhomboids

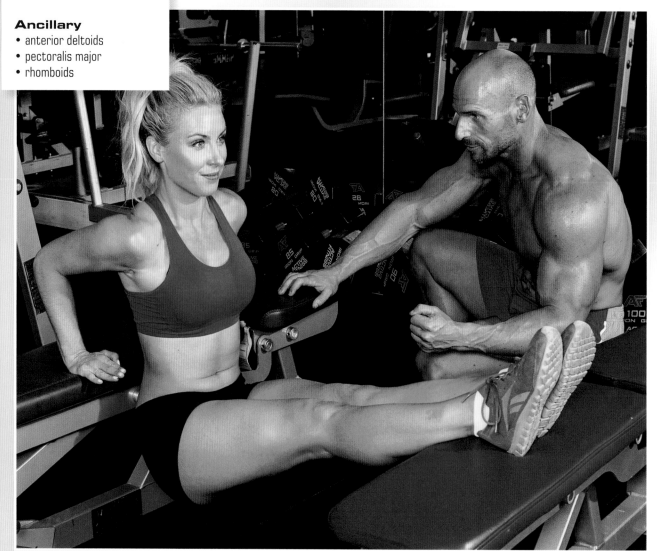

PROPER FORM
Do it right
- Perform controlled repetitions.
- Keep your upper body straight and your torso stabilized.
- Lower yourself until your upper arms are parallel to the ground.

Avoid
- Excessive speed.
- Shallow or bouncy repetitions.
- An unsteady hand placement.

MODIFICATIONS
Beginner
- Keep your heels planted on the ground.

Advanced
- Place a barbell plate on your thighs to add greater resistance.

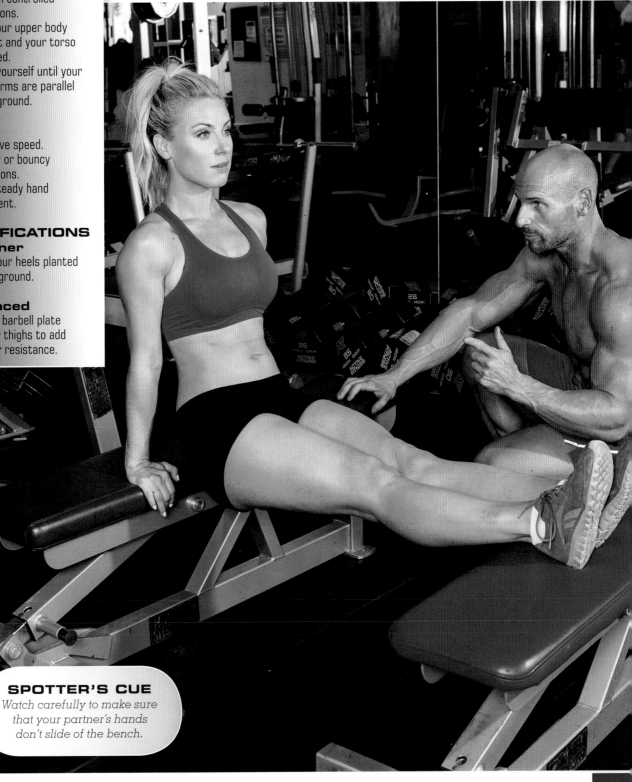

SPOTTER'S CUE
Watch carefully to make sure that your partner's hands don't slide of the bench.

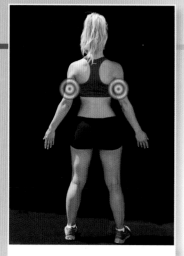

OVERHEAD ROPE EXTENSION

1 Using a rope attachment on the lower part of a cable machine, stand with your back to the cable stack. With an overhand grip, firmly grasp the rope, bending your arms back to roughly a 90-degree angle with your elbows tucked in toward your ears.

2 Extend your forearms upward while keeping the rope together until your arms are nearly locked out overhead.

3 Lower, and repeat for 10 to 12 repetitions.

MUSCLE ACTION
Primary
• triceps brachii

Ancillary
• anterior deltoids
• pectoralis major
• rhomboids

SPOTTER'S CUE
Assist at the forearms or rope attachment to help raise the weight and to keep the arms positioned correctly.

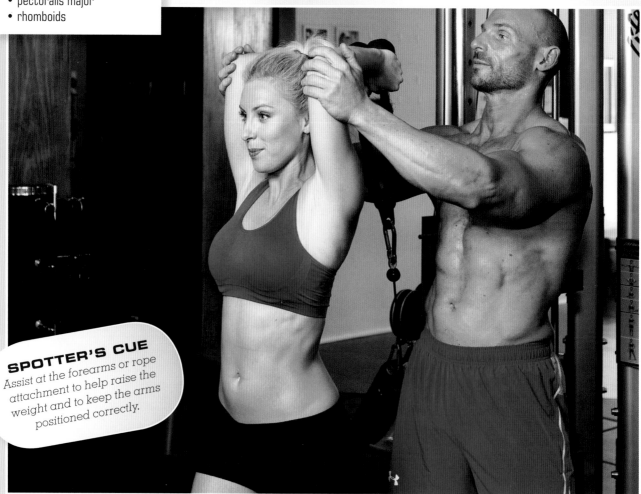

PROPER FORM
Do it right
- Have your training partner hand you the cable once you are positioned in front of the cable machine.
- Hold your upper arms stationary throughout.
- Extend directly above your head.

Avoid
- Allowing your elbows to flare outward.
- Extending to full lockout—you want to keep the tension on your triceps and off your elbow joints.
- Leaning backward.

MODIFICATIONS
Beginner
- Use a dumbbell.

Advanced
- Use one arm at a time.

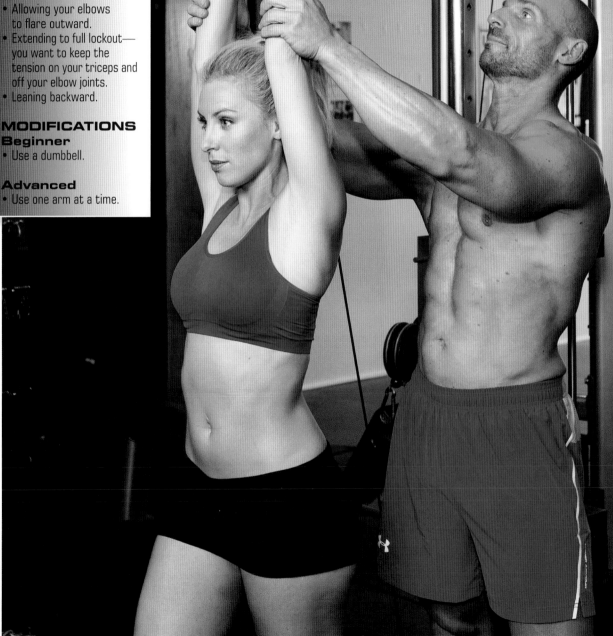

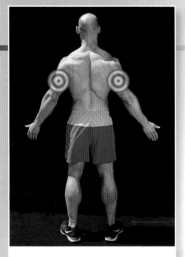

REVERSE-GRIP PUSHDOWN

1 Using a short bar attached to the top of a cable machine, stand facing the cable stack. With an underhand grip, grasp the bar attachment, bending your forearms up while keeping your elbows tucked in at your sides.

2 Extend the bar straight down to full extension.

3 Return, and repeat for 10 to 15 repetitions.

MUSCLE ACTION
Primary
- triceps brachii

Ancillary
- anterior deltoids
- pectoralis major
- rhomboids

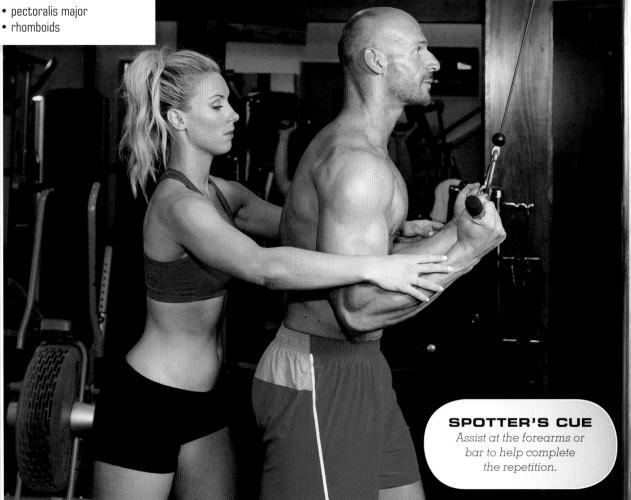

SPOTTER'S CUE
Assist at the forearms or bar to help complete the repetition.

PROPER FORM
Do it right
- Perform slow and controlled repetitions.
- Hold your upper arms stationary throughout.
- Move through a full and controlled range of motion.

Avoid
- Excessive speed.
- An incomplete range of motion.
- Allowing your elbows to flare outward.

MODIFICATIONS
Beginner
- Use an overhand grip.

Advanced
- Use one arm at a time.

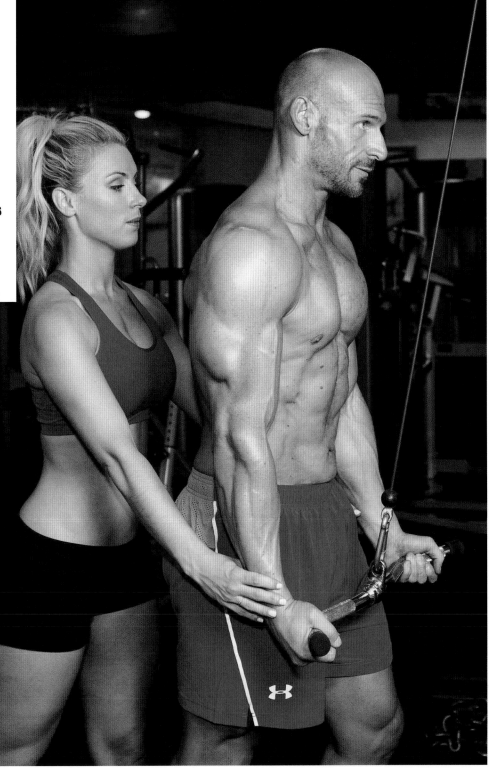

REVERSE CRUNCH

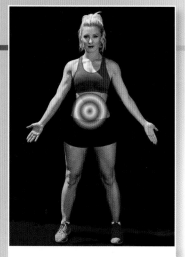

1 Lie back on a flat bench with your knees bent. Bring your feet up, allowing them to dangle. Place your hands behind you, and grasp the bench pad.

2 Raise your legs both back and up, while keeping a tucked-in position, so that your knees travel both backward and vertically.

3 Return to the starting position, and repeat for 15 to 20 repetitions.

MUSCLE ACTION
Primary
- rectus abdominis
- obliques

Ancillary
- erector spinae
- hip flexors

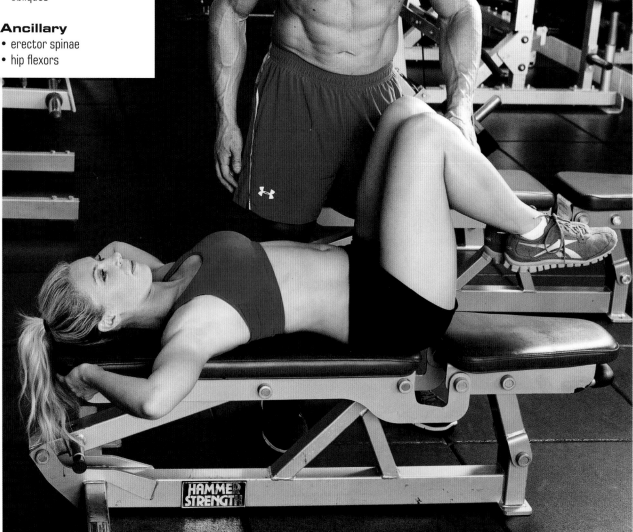

PROPER FORM
Do it right
- Keep your legs bent throughout.
- Contract your abs at the top of the movement.
- Move through a full and controlled range of motion.

Avoid
- Excessive speed.
- An incomplete range of motion.
- Letting go of the bench.

MODIFICATIONS
Beginner
- Perform fewer repetitions.

Advanced
- Grasp a Swiss ball between your thighs.

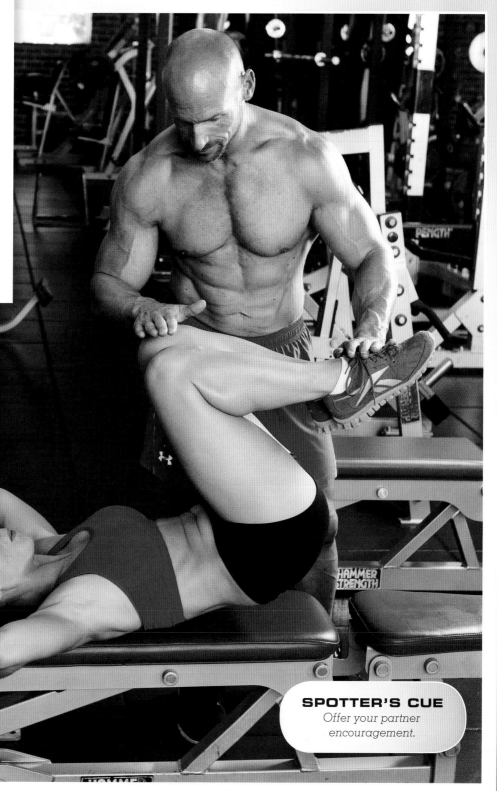

SPOTTER'S CUE
Offer your partner encouragement.

TWISTING CRUNCH

1 Lie back on a flat bench with your knees bent. Bring your feet up, allowing them to dangle. Place your palms on your temples near your ears.

2 Raise your torso toward your knees, and bring one elbow toward the opposite knee.

3 Lower, and alternate sides for 15 to 20 repetitions per side.

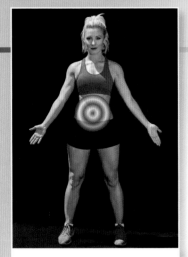

MUSCLE ACTION
Primary
- rectus abdominis
- obliques

Ancillary
- erector spinae

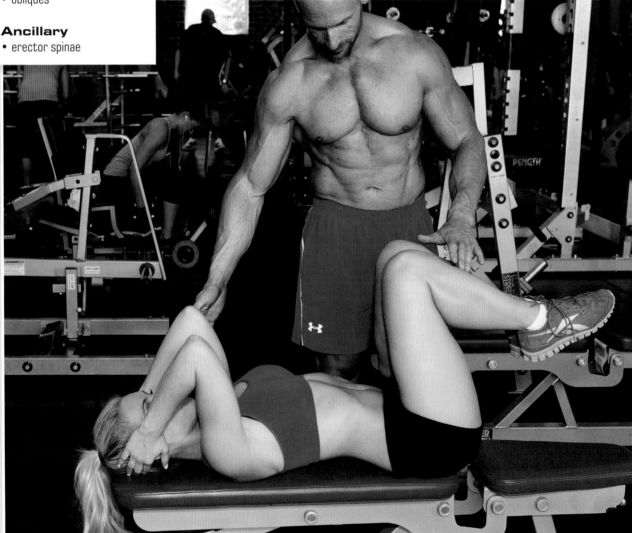

PROPER FORM
Do it right
- Lead as if pulling from your belly button.
- Contract your abs at the top of the movement.
- Keep your torso stabilized.

Avoid
- Using your neck.
- Speedy repetitions.
- Lifting your lower back off the bench.

MODIFICATIONS
Beginner
- Keep your feet planted on the bench.

Advanced
- Hold a barbell plate on your chest.

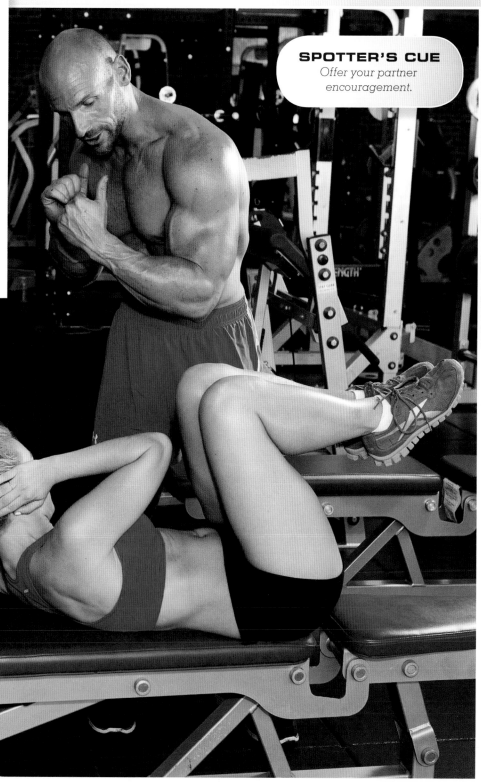

SPOTTER'S CUE
Offer your partner encouragement.

PARTNER STRETCHES

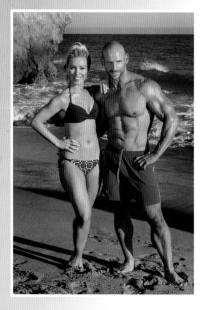

You've probably seen scores of stretches out there that target just about every body part. Some trainers say to perform them before you exercise, and others say it is best after (including me). So you may ask yourself, "Why stretch *after* exercising?" Well, you will probably experience muscle soreness after a hard workout. Stretching can relieve the pain, and it increases blood flow to those sore muscles. This facilitates the removal of waste products produced by tissue damage and encourages muscle repair and growth.

The following stretches can be done in the gym, on the beach, indoors, outdoors—just about anywhere. You can perform them both during your workout and especially following your resistance training for the day. Their proper placement can be found in chapter 6, with each stretch corresponding to the muscles worked for that particular day. You can also perform them consecutively as a single circuit. Hold each stretch for the prescribed amount of time in a static, or held, position. Then, switch roles and have your partner perform the stretch on you.

Although often neglected and commonly viewed as one of the less "glamorous" portions of one's transformation, stretching is imperative—if for nothing else than to help alleviate aches and pains, remove toxins and, most especially, work through a full and complete range of motion. Exercising with full integrity and form will allow you to develop more lean muscle tissue, which is one of your main goals in attaining your complete physique.

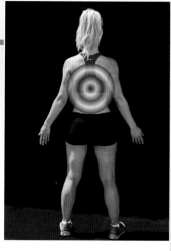

PARTNER SURRENDER STRETCH

1 Sit with your legs apart facing your partner in the same position.

2 With your feet touching and holding your partner's wrists, lean back while pulling forward until your partner's arms and torso are fully extended toward you.

3 Hold for 10 to 30 seconds, and then switch roles.

MUSCLE ACTION
- latissimus dorsi
- erector spinae

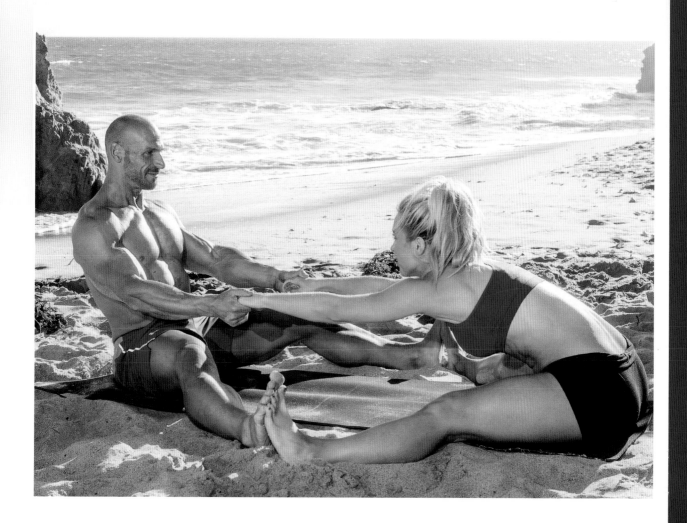

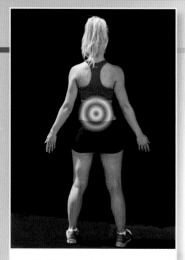

MUSCLE ACTION
• erector spinae

LOWER-BACK STRETCH

1 Have your partner lie in a supine position. Place one hand by a knee and the other on the opposite shoulder, and then bend the leg.

2 Your partner should keep his or her shoulders close to the ground as you gently rotate the bent leg to the side until it touches or nearly touches the ground.

3 Hold for 10 to 15 seconds, and then perform on the other side. Switch roles, and repeat.

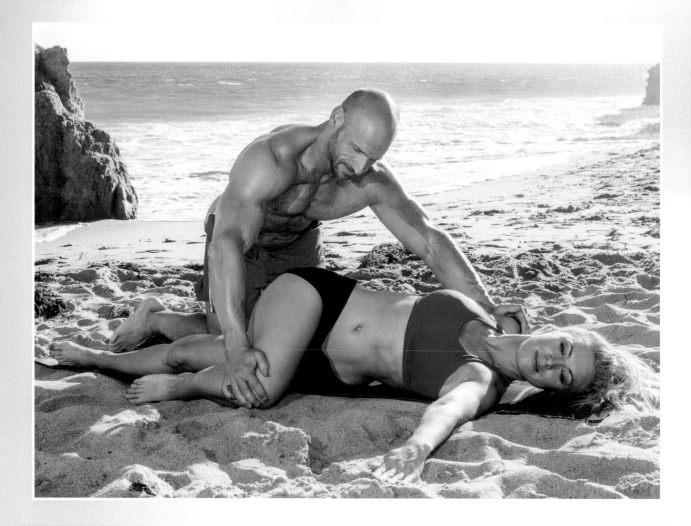

CHEST STRETCH

1 Have your partner seated while you position yourself behind on bent knees. Your partner's hands should be behind his or her head with fingers interlocked.

2 Gently hold at the elbows, and pull outward so as to open your partner's chest.

3 Hold for 10 to 30 seconds, and then switch roles.

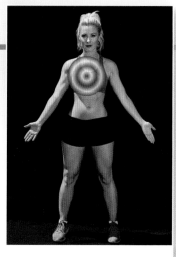

MUSCLE ACTION
• pectorals

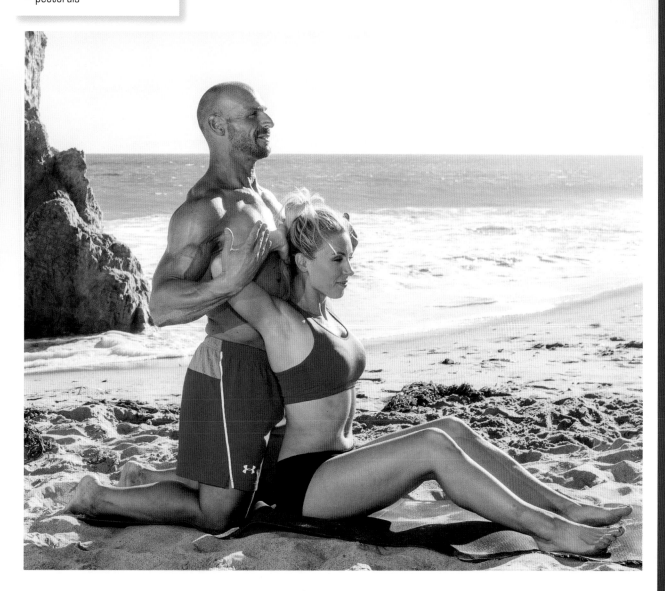

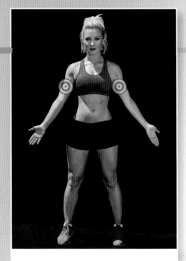

MUSCLE ACTION
• biceps brachii

BICEPS STRETCH

1 Have your partner seated while you position yourself behind him or her on bent knees. Your partner's arms should be extended out to each side.

2 Gently hold your partner's hands and pull outward and back until his or her arms are nearly straight.

3 Hold for 10 to 30 seconds, and then switch roles.

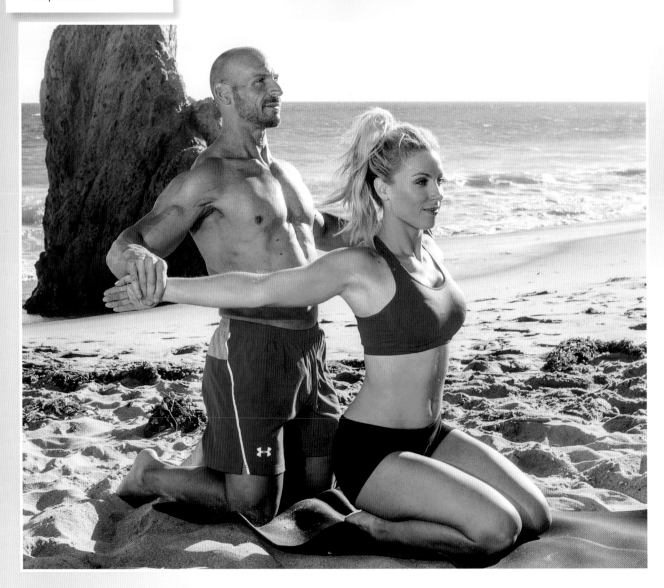

QUAD STRETCH

1 Have your partner lay on his or her side with one forearm planted on the ground and the other hand in front and legs stacked atop each other.

2 Gently hold just above the knee and the toes as you bend the top leg backward at the knee while simultaneously pulling the leg back to accentuate the stretch.

3 Hold for 10 to 30 seconds per leg, and then switch roles.

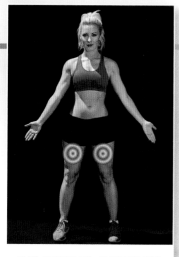

MUSCLE ACTION
- rectus femoris
- vastus lateralis
- vastus intermedius
- vastus medialis

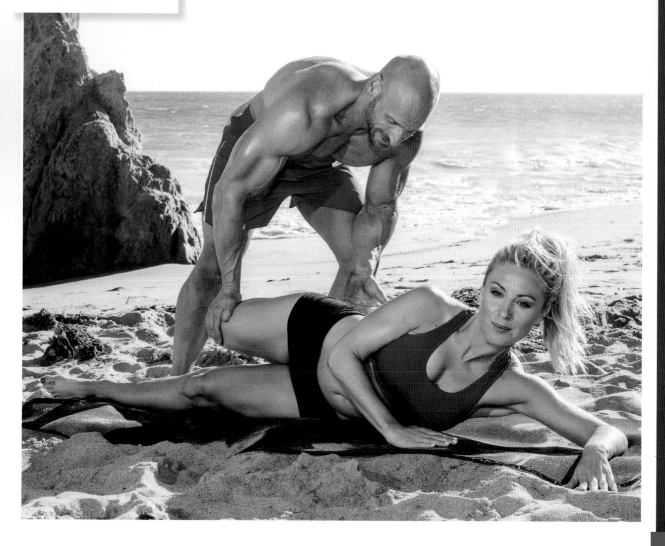

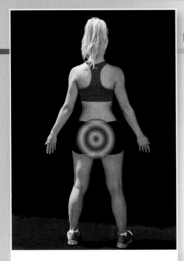

MUSCLE ACTION
- gluteus medius
- piriformis

GLUTE/GROIN STRETCH

1 Have your partner lie in a supine position with both arms at the sides and legs straight.

2 With one hand placed just below the knee and the other on the ankle, gently bend one leg at the knee.

3 Lean in as you move the leg back and to the side.

4 Hold for 10 to 30 seconds per leg, and then switch roles.

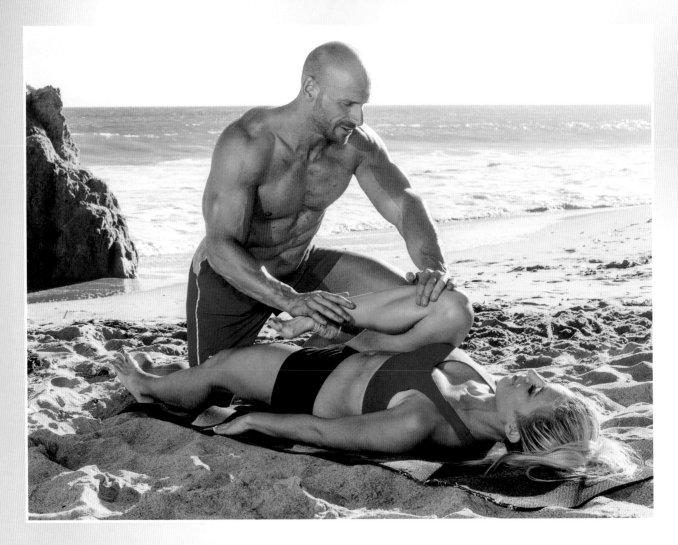

HAMSTRINGS STRETCH

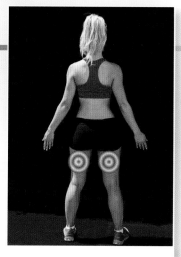

MUSCLE ACTION
- biceps femoris
- semitendinosus
- semimembranosus

1 Have your partner lie in a supine position with both arms at the sides and legs straight.

2 While placing one hand gently on his or her thigh for support, gently hold the other leg by the ankle and raise it straight up to a 90-degree angle.

3 Hold for 10 to 30 seconds per leg, and then switch roles.

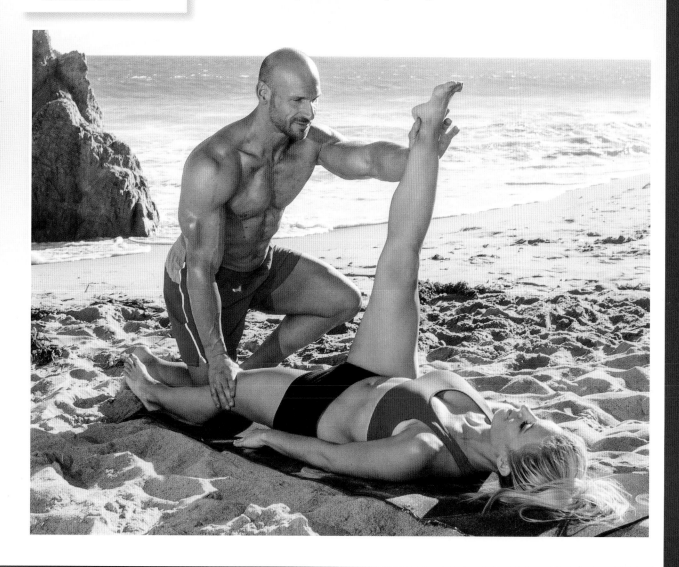

CALF STRETCH

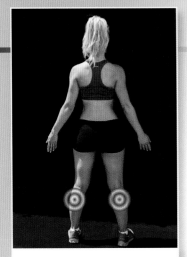

MUSCLE ACTION
- gastrocnemius
- soleus

1 Have your partner lie in a supine position with both arms at the sides and legs straight.

2 Gently hold one leg by the ankle and raise it straight up to a 90-degree angle while placing your other hand on the top of the foot and lightly pushing downward to accentuate the stretch.

3 Hold for 10 to 30 seconds per calf, and then switch roles.

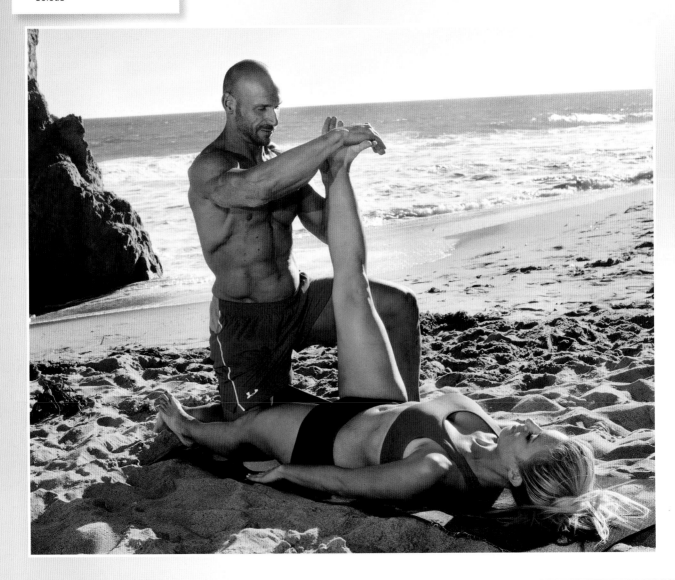

DELTOID STRETCH

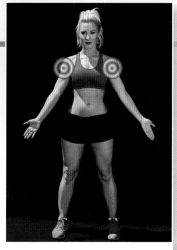

1 Have your partner seated while you position yourself behind him or her on bent knees.

2 Place your hand on one shoulder as you gently pull the same-sided arm across the front of his or her torso, being sure to keep the shoulder down and the torso straight on.

3 Hold for 10 to 30 seconds per shoulder, and then switch roles.

MUSCLE ACTION
- anterior deltoids
- medial deltoids
- posterior deltoids

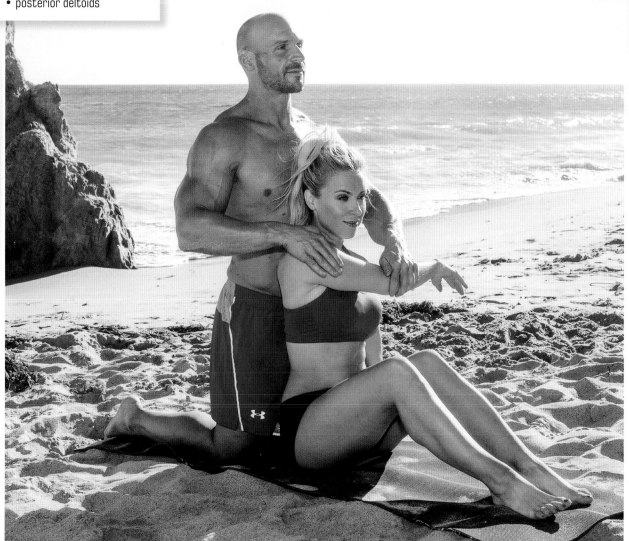

NECK STRETCH

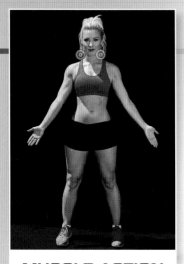

MUSCLE ACTION
• sternocleidomastoid

1 Have your partner seated while you position yourself behind him or her on bent knees.

2 Place a hand on one shoulder as you place your other hand on his or her head and gently tilt your partner's neck to the side, being sure to apply minimal pressure.

3 Hold for 10 to 30 seconds per side, and then switch roles.

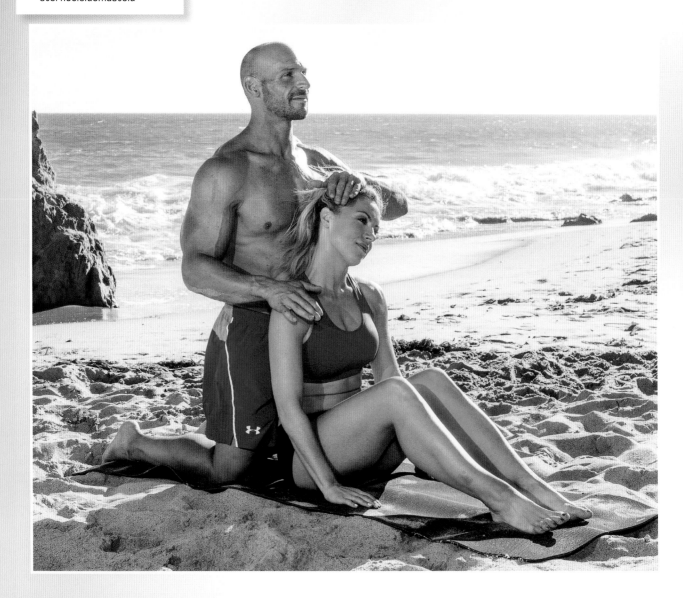

TRICEPS STRETCH

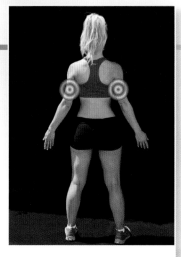

1 Have your partner seated while you position yourself behind him or her on bent knees.

2 Holding at the elbow and hand, raise one arm above his or her head, and bend. Gently pull the arm closed to accentuate the stretch.

3 Hold for 10 to 30 seconds per arm, and then switch roles.

MUSCLE ACTION
• triceps brachii

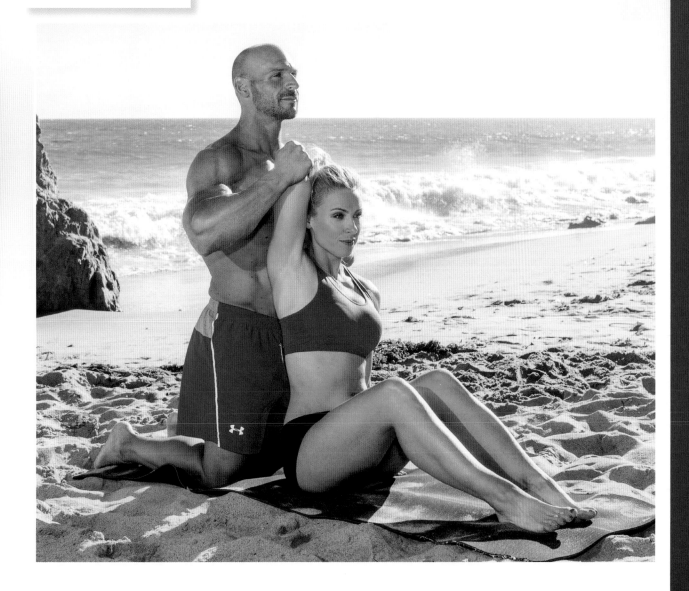

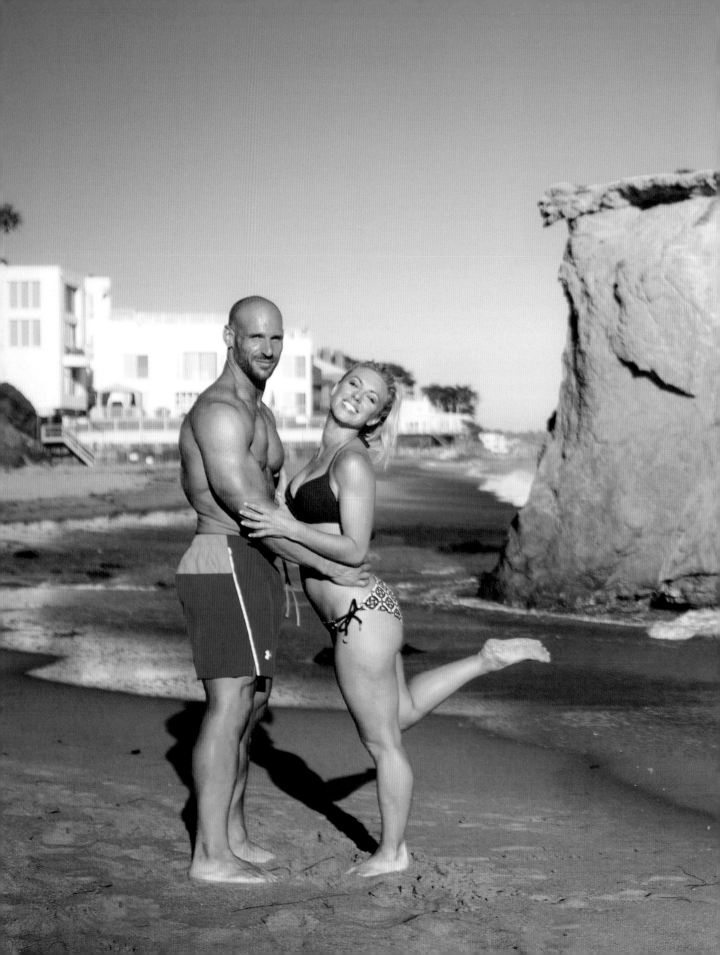

7 THE PORTABLE WORKOUT

What do you do when you can't make it to the gym? Are you traveling on a business trip or a family vacation and have no access to traditional gym equipment? Maybe you just need a break from the gym workouts and need to try something different that focuses more on overall body toning and conditioning. Well, you can still get your workout in, whether you do it in your backyard, on a beach or just about anywhere. Portability is key—all you'll need are resistance bands and a Swiss Ball, both affordable and fully functional.

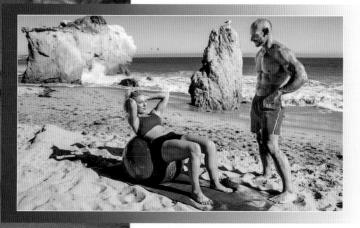
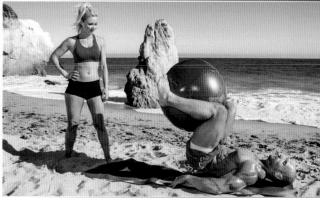

NO EXCUSES

Your transformation can only occur when you've deemed it a need. Let's be realistic—if you waited until the perfect time to start your fitness program and for the planets to align, you'd never start at all. Far too often potential clients tell me, "Hollis I hear you, and I am onboard . . . I just can't start right now."

There are so many excuses for the delay but when I ask why, I so often hear something like "I am on the road so much or I just booked my vacation." And I say "So what!" There's not a gym available where you're going or a healthy food choice in that town? Let me be very clear here: There is no tomorrow, there is only today. Start now.

Consider that professional bodybuilders and other athletes derive their income from their bodies, and they travel extensively. In fact, the top pros travel globally and are often expected to not only show up in decent shape but also expected to improve upon their physiques (come contest time). They find a way to train and get their clean meals in on the road constantly and consistently. If they can do this, there's no excuse for the rest of us. None.

COMING FULL CIRCLE

The Portable Workout features three circuits of exercises that provide you with a full-body workout.

CIRCUIT 1
- Band Resisted Push-Up
- Bent-Over One-Arm Band Row
- Upright Band Row
- Front Shoulder Band Raise
- Lateral Band Raise

Perform all five exercises, and then rest for 45 to 60 seconds. Repeat three times, and then move on to Circuit 2.

CIRCUIT 2
- Band Overhead Triceps Extension
- Alternating Band Curl
- Band Squat
- Band Lunge

Perform all four exercises, and then rest for 45 to 60 seconds. Repeat three times, and then move on to Circuit 3.

CIRCUIT 3
- Swiss Ball Crunch
- Swiss Ball Reverse Crunch
- Swiss Ball Rollout
- Swiss Ball Hip Crossover

Perform all four exercises, and then rest for 45 to 60 seconds. Repeat two times, and you have concluded.

IT'S JUST A MATTER OF TIME

Getting into shape does not really demand a heavy investment in time. At its most demanding, the *Complete Physique* program calls for performing 4 hours of resistance training per week and 200 minutes of cardiovascular activity. It simply comes down to when that work is performed. Whether it's before, during or after work, we all share the same 24-hour time frame. It doesn't matter when. It doesn't even matter where. Just get it done. Do the work.

TAKE IT OUTSIDE

Another important reason for this chapter is the very real fact that some people just aren't comfortable working out in the gym. To me, the gym is the great equalizer. It doesn't matter if you're sporting six-pack abs or are out of shape and obese. Rich or poor. Within its walls, you still have to do the work—and that is perhaps the gym's most compelling attribute. You can't pay for the work to be done for you. You yourself have to take action, regardless of who you are. The gym reveals the inner workings of what you are.

Still, your transformational process doesn't have to be limited to the confines of a gym's walls. You can easily set up and work out outside them, too. I'm confident that you don't ever have to step inside a gym or other fitness center to claim the body of your dreams. To say, "This is the only way to see results," simply isn't true. There are multiple routes to any destination. So in the end, if exercising in private rather than among a crowd makes the difference between getting it done and not getting it done, then go for it wherever you feel most comfortable.

You can perform the Portable Workout just about anywhere from your backyard to the beach—or even in a hotel room. It features a baker's dozen of efficient exercises that are divided into three circuits. Simply perform all the exercises in each circuit for the prescribed number of repetitions back to back, trying to keep your rest between circuits down to 45 to 60 seconds for an increased challenge.

The only equipment you'll need is a Swiss Ball and stretchable resistance exercise bands (when traveling, just deflate the ball, and you'll still have room in your bag for trail mix, a protein bar or shaker bottle to keep fueled for performance). The bands, which often come with handles, offer convenient change, coming in a variety of resistance levels, so that you can keep steadily progressing as your conditioning improves.

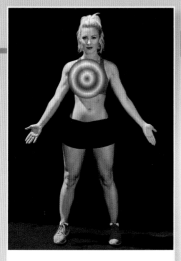

BAND RESISTED PUSH-UP

1 Place a resistance band around the rear of your shoulders and running down your arms, and place your hands shoulder-width apart on the ground.

2 Position yourself on your toes with your body in an elongated position.

3 Lower your chest nearly to the ground by bending your elbows while keeping your chest directly above your hands, feeling the added tension from the band. Repeat for 12 to 15 repetitions.

MUSCLE ACTION
Primary
- pectoralis major

Ancillary
- anterior deltoids
- rhomboids
- triceps brachii
- rectus abdominis
- erector spinae

PROPER FORM
Do it right
- Firmly grasp the bands.
- Keep your upper body straight and your torso stabilized.
- Lower yourself until your upper arms are parallel to the ground.

Avoid
- Excessive speed.
- Shallow or bouncy repetitions.
- Allowing the lower back to dip too far.

MODIFICATIONS
Beginner
- A wider hand spacing will decrease the range of motion.

Advanced
- Raise one leg.

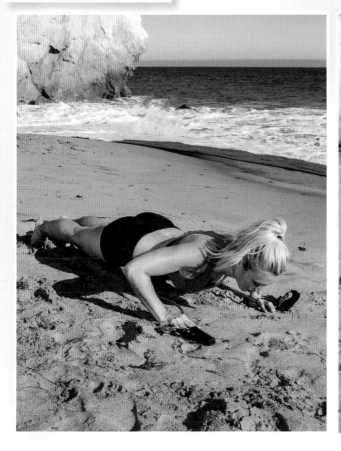

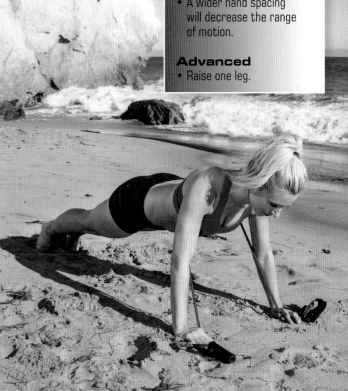

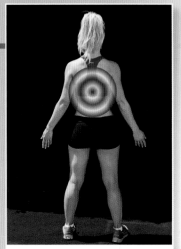

BENT-OVER ONE-ARM BAND ROW

1 Stand while holding one end of a resistance band in one hand, and step firmly on the other end of the band with the opposite foot, leaving a little slack.

2 Lean forward until your torso is parallel to the ground, while placing your free hand on your thigh for support and extending your opposite leg behind you.

2 Pull both up and back, until your hand nearly touches your chest.

3 Lower, and repeat for 12 to 15 repetitions per arm.

MUSCLE ACTION
Primary
- latissimus dorsi
- trapezius
- rhomboids

Ancillary
- biceps brachii
- rear deltoids
- rectus abdominis
- obliques
- erector spinae
- forearm extensors
- forearm flexors

PROPER FORM
Do it right
- Look for a full contraction at the top.
- Stabilize your torso.
- Move through a fluid range of motion.

Avoid
- Rounding your back.
- Not stepping firmly on the band.
- Excessive speed.

MODIFICATIONS
Beginner
- Use a lighter resistance.

Advanced
- Raise one leg.

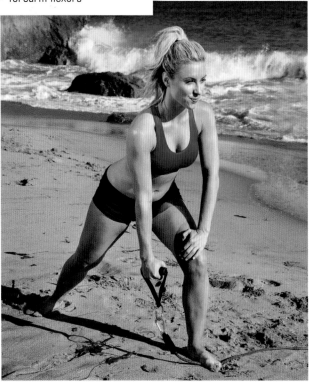

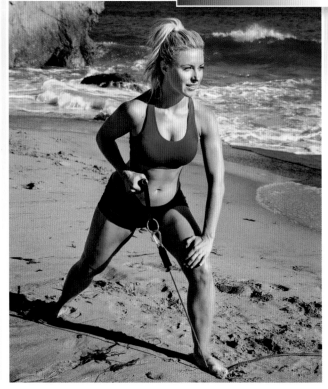

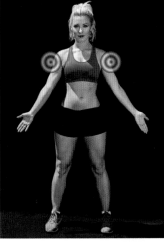

UPRIGHT BAND ROW

1 Firmly stand on a resistance band with both feet while holding the handles with an overhand close grip with your arms extended downward.

2 With your elbows leading, raise your arms upward, keeping your hands and the band close to your body.

3 Lower, and repeat for 12 to 15 repetitions.

MUSCLE ACTION
Primary
• medial deltoids

Ancillary
• trapezius
• rhomboids
• forearm extensors
• forearm flexors

PROPER FORM
Do it right
• Keep the band close to your body.
• Lead with your elbows.
• Raise your hands to chin level.

Avoid
• Dropping your elbows.
• Lifting the bands too far from your body.
• Excessive speed or momentum.

MODIFICATIONS
Beginner
• Alternate arms.

Advanced
• Use a heavier resistance.

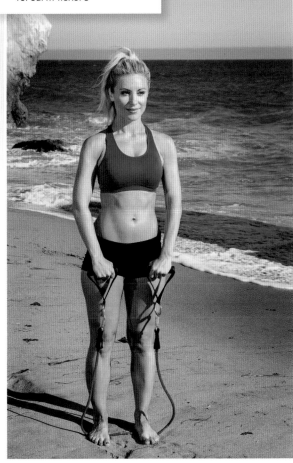

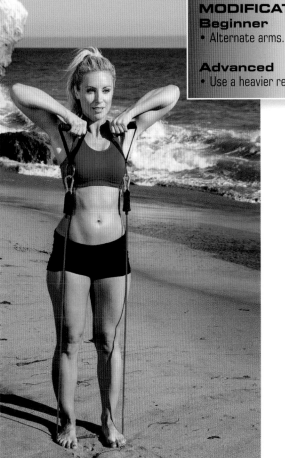

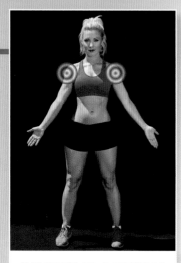

FRONT SHOULDER BAND RAISE

1 Firmly stand on a resistance band with both feet while holding the handles with an overhand shoulder-width grip with your arms extended downward.

2 Raise both arms straight up until they are parallel to the ground, maintaining a very slight bend in your arms and keeping your palms facing downward.

3 Lower, and repeat for 12 to 15 repetitions.

MUSCLE ACTION
Primary
- anterior deltoids

Ancillary
- trapezius
- rhomboids
- forearm extensors
- forearm flexors

PROPER FORM
Do it right
- Maintain an erect posture throughout.
- Keep your arms slightly bent.
- Raise your arms parallel to the ground.

Avoid
- Keeping your arms completely straight.
- Not stepping firmly on the band.
- Excessive speed or momentum.

MODIFICATIONS
Beginner
- Use a lighter resistance.

Advanced
- Use one arm at a time.

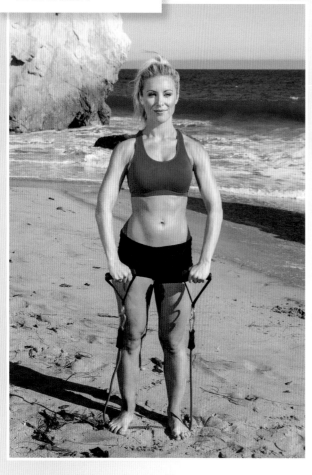
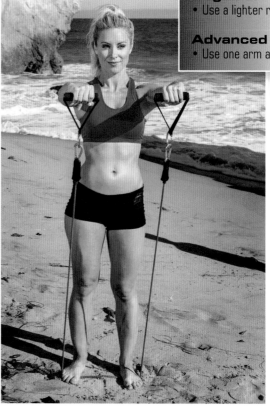

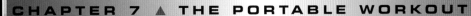

LATERAL BAND RAISE

1 Firmly stand on a resistance band with both feet while holding the handles at your sides with your arms extended downward.

2 With a slight bend in your elbows, pull your arms directly out to the sides, following an arced pathway, until they are parallel to the ground.

3 Lower, and repeat for 12 to 15 repetitions.

MUSCLE ACTION
Primary
- medial deltoids

Ancillary
- trapezius
- rhomboids
- forearm extensors
- forearm flexors

PROPER FORM
Do it right
- Maintain an erect posture throughout.
- Keep your arms slightly bent.
- Point your thumbs slightly downward as you raise your arms.

Avoid
- Raising your arms above parallel to the ground.
- Not stepping firmly on the band.
- Excessive speed or momentum.

MODIFICATIONS
Beginner
- Use a lighter resistance.

Advanced
- Alternate arms.

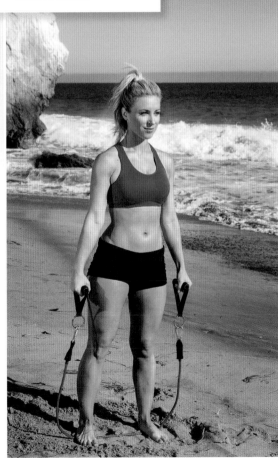

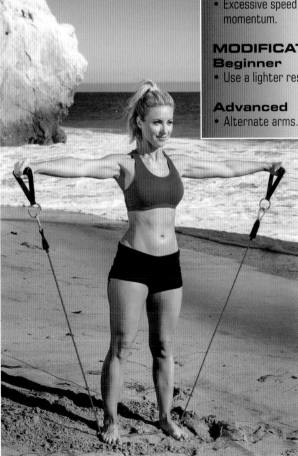

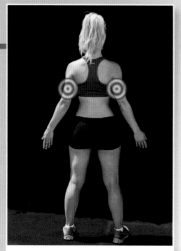

BAND OVERHEAD TRICEPS EXTENSION

1 Kneel on the ground with a band running firmly just below your knees.

2 With a handle in each hand, raise your arms up with your elbows in and your forearms bent behind your head running parallel to your lower legs.

3 Raise your forearms straight up to full overhead extension.

4 Lower, and repeat for 12 to 15 repetitions.

MUSCLE ACTION
Primary
- triceps brachii

Ancillary
- rhomboids
- rectus abdominis
- erector spinae

PROPER FORM
Do it right
- Keep your elbows locked in.
- Extend directly above your head.
- Maintain an erect posture throughout.

Avoid
- Allowing your elbows to flare outward.
- Extending forward rather than straight up.
- Leaning backward.

MODIFICATIONS
Beginner
- Use a lighter resistance.

Advanced
- Use one arm at a time.

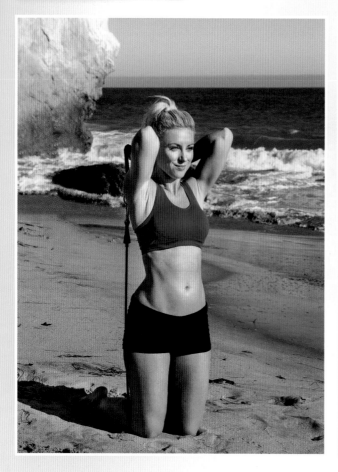

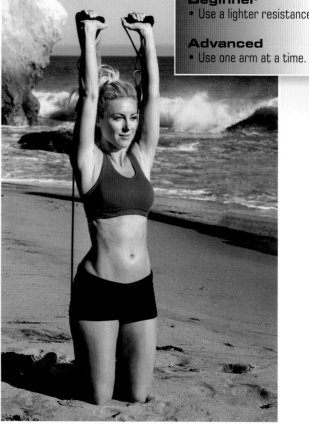

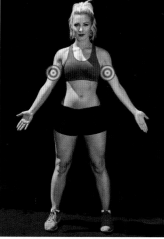

ALTERNATING BAND CURL

1 Firmly stand on a resistance band with both feet while holding the handles with an underhand grip approximately shoulder-width apart with your arms extended downward.

2 Bend your elbow, one arm at a time, as you curl the weight up toward your shoulder in an arced pathway.

3 Lower, and repeat with the other arm. Perform 12 to 15 repetitions per arm.

MUSCLE ACTION
Primary
- biceps brachii

Ancillary
- forearm extensors
- forearm flexors
- rectus abdominis
- erector spinae

PROPER FORM
Do it right
- Move through a full and controlled range of motion.
- Keep your elbows close to your body throughout.
- Move one arm at a time.

Avoid
- Using momentum to swing the resistance upward.
- An incomplete range of motion.
- Excessively involving your lower back to drive the movement.

MODIFICATIONS
Beginner
- Use both arms simultaneously.

Advanced
- Use a neutral grip, moving your hands in a hammer-like motion.

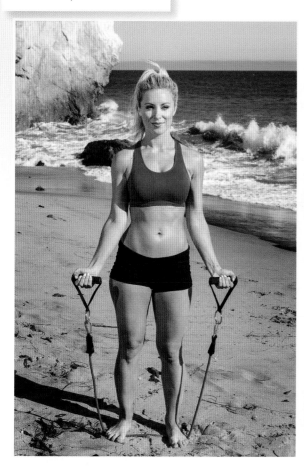

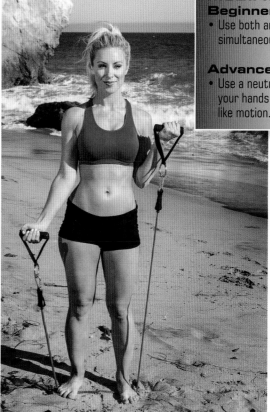

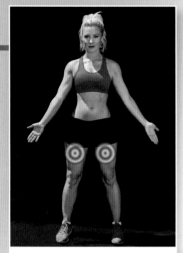

BAND SQUAT

1 Firmly stand on a resistance band with your feet apart in shoulder-width stance with your toes straight-on and your knees soft or slightly bent. Hold the handles of the band by your shoulders with your palms facing forward.

2 Bend your knees, lowering yourself until your thighs are parallel to the ground while keeping an erect posture.

3 Push through your heels to return to the starting position, and then repeat for 12 to 15 repetitions.

MUSCLE ACTION
Primary
- rectus femoris
- vastus lateralis
- vastus intermedius
- vastus medialis
- gluteus maximus
- biceps femoris
- semitendinosus
- semimembranosus

Ancillary
- erector spinae
- rectus abdominis
- adductor magnus
- soleus
- gastrocnemius

PROPER FORM
Do it right
- Squat until your thighs are parallel to the ground.
- Keep your hands close to your shoulders.
- Push through your heels to drive the movement.

Avoid
- Hyperextending your toes past your feet.
- Allowing the arms to flair away from your shoulders.
- Pushing through your toes to drive the movement.

MODIFICATIONS
Beginner
- A wider stance will decrease the range of motion.

Advanced
- A closer stance will increase the range of motion.

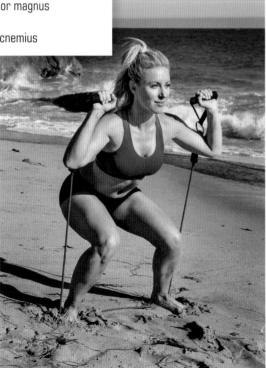

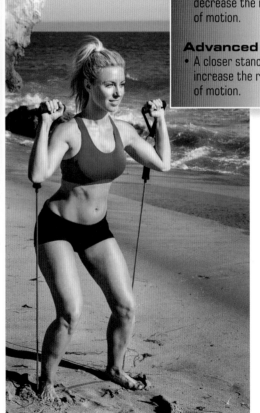

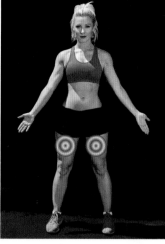

BAND LUNGE

1 Step firmly on a band with one foot while holding the handles by your shoulders with your palms facing each other. Move into in a staggered stance with one foot on the band placed flat on the ground in front of you and the other foot behind you resting on your toes.

2 Keeping your back straight, drop your back knee while simultaneously bending your front leg until your front thigh is parallel to the ground.

3 Push through your front heel to raise yourself to full extension. Repeat for 12 to 15 repetitions per leg.

MUSCLE ACTION
Primary
- rectus femoris
- vastus lateralis
- vastus intermedius
- vastus medialis
- gluteus maximus
- biceps femoris
- semitendinosus
- semimembranosus

Ancillary
- erector spinae
- rectus abdominis
- adductor magnus
- soleus
- gastrocnemius

PROPER FORM
Do it right
- Push through the front heel to drive the movement.
- Keep your hands close to your shoulders.
- Lunge only until your front thigh is parallel to the ground.

Avoid
- Allowing your knee to hyperextend past your front foot.
- Allowing your arms to flair away from your shoulders.
- Pushing through your toe to drive the movement.

MODIFICATIONS
Beginner
- Use a lighter resistance.

Advanced
- Use a heavier resistance.

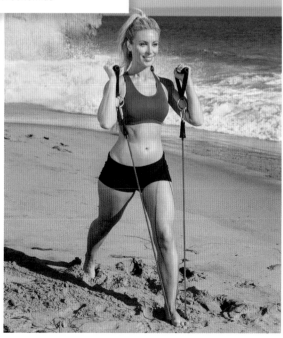

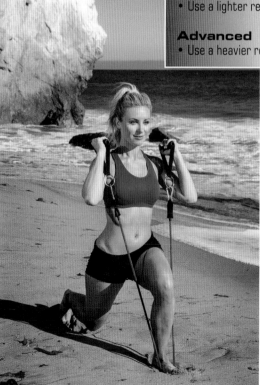

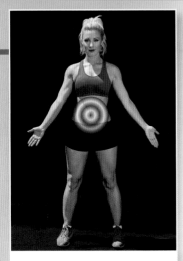

SWISS BALL CRUNCH

1 Lie on your back on a Swiss ball with your legs bent, your shoulders supported on the ball and your palms on your ears.

2 Raise your torso toward your knees.

3 Lower, and repeat for 15 to 20 repetitions.

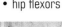

MUSCLE ACTION
Primary
- rectus abdominis
- transversus abdominis
- obliques

Ancillary
- erector spinae
- hip flexors

PROPER FORM
Do it right
- Keep your legs bent throughout.
- Contract your abs at the top of the movement.
- Move through a full and controlled range of motion.

Avoid
- Excessive speed.
- An incomplete range of motion.
- Wobbling on the ball.

MODIFICATIONS
Beginner
- Perform this exercise on the ground.

Advanced
- Twist to alternating sides as you rise up.

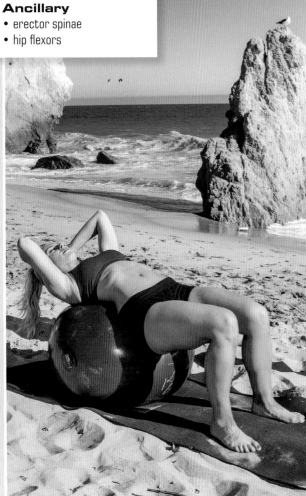

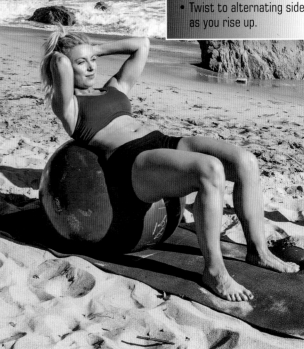

SWISS BALL REVERSE CRUNCH

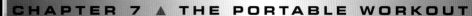

1 Lie on your back on the ground with your arms at your sides and your legs bent and straddling a Swiss ball.

2 Raise your legs both back and up, while keeping a tucked-in position, so that your knees travel both backward and vertically.

3 Return to the starting position, and repeat for 15 to 20 repetitions.

MUSCLE ACTION
Primary
- rectus abdominis
- transversus abdominis
- obliques

Ancillary
- erector spinae
- hip flexors

PROPER FORM
Do it right
- Keep your legs bent.
- Hold the ball firmly in place.
- Move through a full and controlled range of motion.

Avoid
- Excessive speed.
- Lifting your head.
- An incomplete range of motion.

MODIFICATIONS
Beginner
- Perform this exercise without the ball.

Advanced
- Straighten your legs.

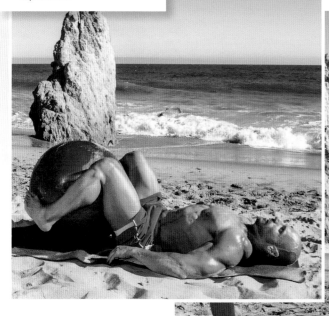

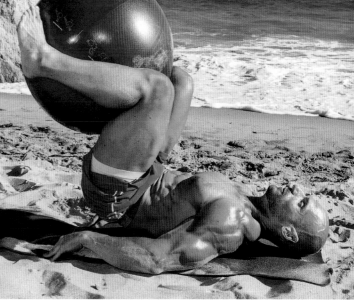

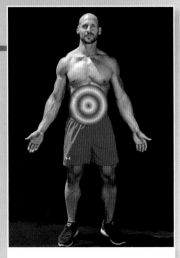

SWISS BALL ROLLOUT

1 Kneel behind a Swiss ball, and place your fists on top.

2 Remaining on your knees with your back straight, roll the ball forward, leading with your arms and following through with your entire body.

3 Roll back using the same range of motion while keeping an erect posture.

4 Repeat for 15 to 20 repetitions.

MUSCLE ACTION
Primary
- rectus abdominis
- transversus abdominis
- obliques

Ancillary
- erector spinae
- pectoralis major
- rectus femoris

PROPER FORM
Do it right
- Keep your torso elongated throughout.
- Hold the ball firmly in place.
- Move through a full and controlled range of motion.

Avoid
- Excessive speed.
- Allowing your buttocks to lag behind.
- Hyperextending your lower back.

MODIFICATIONS
Beginner
- Perform fewer repetitions.

Advanced
- Roll out side to side.

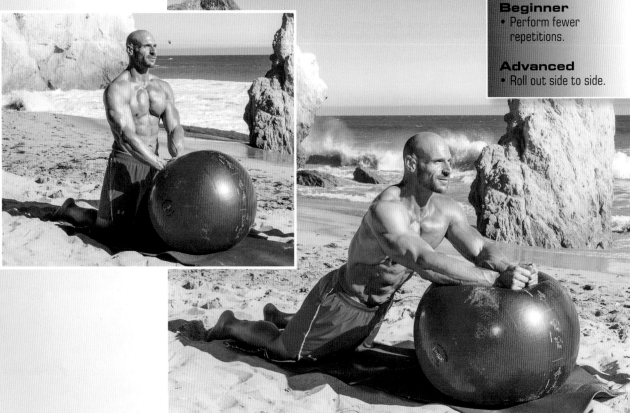

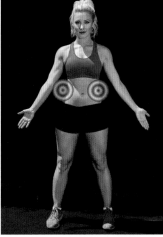

SWISS BALL HIP CROSSOVER

1 Lie on your back on the ground with your arms at your sides. Grip a Swiss ball between your bent legs, lifting it off the ground.

2 Brace your abs as you lower your knees to the side while keeping your torso stabilized, and then reverse to the other direction.

3 Return to the starting position, and repeat for 15 repetitions per side.

MUSCLE ACTION
Primary
• obliques

Ancillary
• erector spinae

PROPER FORM
Do it right
• Keep your legs bent.
• Hold the ball firmly in place.
• Move through a full and controlled range of motion.

Avoid
• Excessive speed.
• Lifting your head.
• Allowing your shoulders to rise off the ground.

MODIFICATIONS
Beginner
• Perform this exercise without the ball.

Advanced
• Straighten your legs.

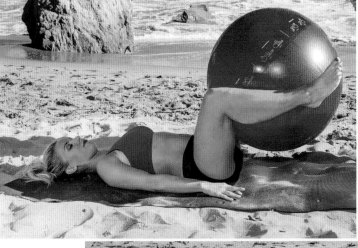

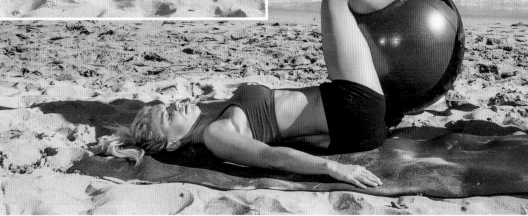

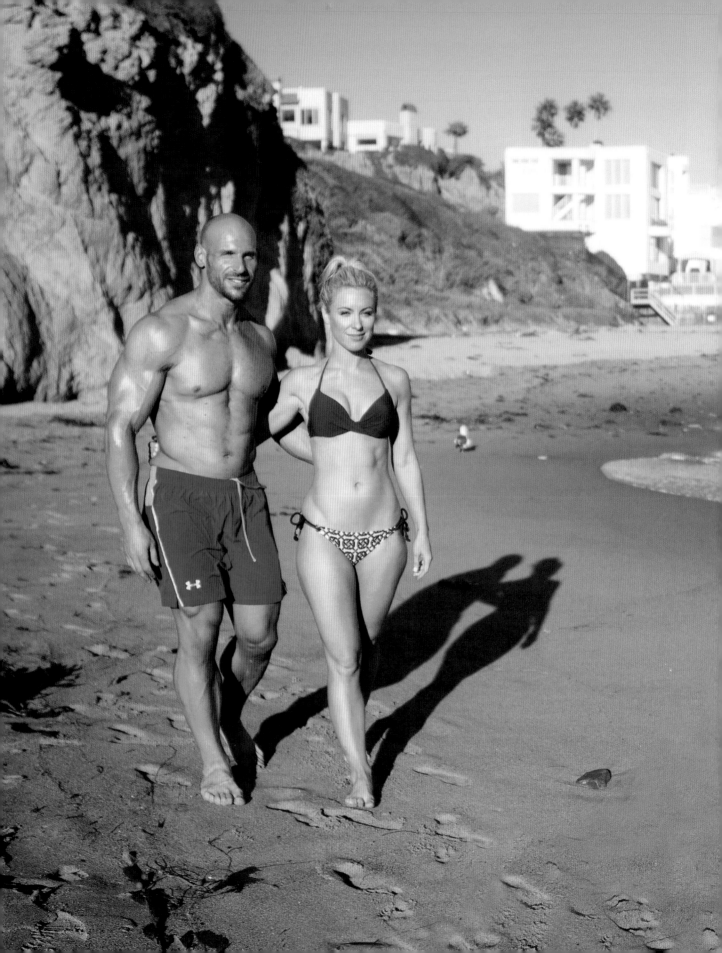

8 THE HUMAN CONDITION

Congratulations, you have either made it through the program or flipped through the book and decided to take part in the #completephysiquechallenge. In either case, it's a win-win situation. One of the main threads in creating this book was journey continuance; the answer to the all-important question, "What's next?" But another major question, its seed planted at the beginning of this volume is "How do you maintain all that you have gained and sacrificed for?"

How do you avoid the rebound effect?

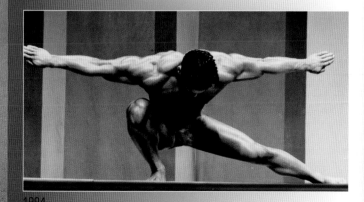

1994

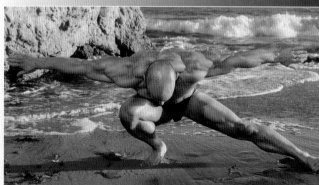

20 years later

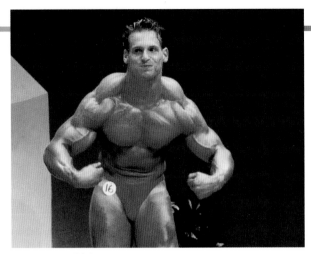

The author in 1994 . . .

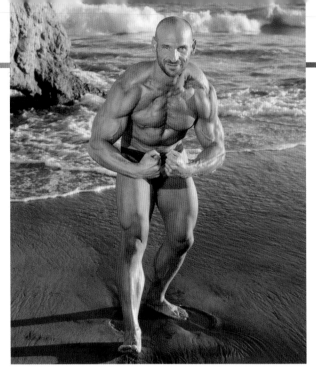

. . . and 20 years later. These photos and those on the previous page show that the *Complete Physique* plan is a lifestyle for the long haul.

As surely as the mindset and intensity of fully committing to any program for 12 weeks cannot be kept up forever—or at least the same level of tenacity—the thought process and physical execution in going forward come down to a few simple words: let up on the gas. What we do know is that muscle will not turn to fat if you stop working out. Your muscle cells will simply shrink, and your fat cells will enlarge and possibly multiply if you ingest more calories than you expend, but this process will reverse itself once you resume healthy eating patterns. Just as we all need a reset button from time to time, sometimes we also need a rest—but not a sleep.

Following principal photography for *Complete Physique*, I allotted myself one week complete rest and recovery from the gym and a relaxed (very relaxed) nutritional regime for that week. That time away gave both my mind and body a much-needed recuperative period, but then I went right back to my healthy lifestyle, keeping myself within striking distance of a complete physique.

This too should be your approach. Get the absolute most out of your 12-week program, and then back off on the throttle just a little bit until you are ready to push it again. Be almost unreasonable in the short term (12 weeks), but realistic over a lifetime. I set my own expectations so high for both books that I had no choice but to achieve because I knew I could scale back once there. I knew that the pictures here of me barely clothed last forever, and, what's more important, I am content in the fact that life cannot and need not be a pedal-to-the-metal kind of pace. Generally speaking, we only build a house once. But we must keep it clean and maintain the outside and pay the utility bills indefinitely in order to keep it running.

THIS WORK IS TIMELESS

As they say in art, it is never finished, so too will you wish to ever-improve your physique. You will never be completely satisfied with the image in the mirror. And therein lies your almost permanent motivation to keep bettering yourself. Keep in mind, however, to not be completely satisfied is not the same as to be dissatisfied. "Dissatisfied" says that this is totally unacceptable. Not being completely satisfied just says you still want more. Wanting more states that this is my best for today, and I look forward to seeing how I can further improve tomorrow.

Back when I was competing in bodybuilding, it was never about beating other athletes, but rather about surpassing my own previous best. The photos on the preceding page and the ones above, taken almost exactly 20 years apart, show that I have kept up my lifestyle and still look to improve. This means not only am I still very much in love with my two life's passions, writing and bodybuilding, but I use periods of time to hit the pedal to improve and then back off to maintain. Remember this is not a sprint, but rather a well-metered marathon.

TO BE HUMAN

Most of us can't help but be curious about the other guy. Whether it is a direct comparison or keeping others in our periphery, to be human is to compare. The images in *Complete Physique* are meant to inspire. They are the result of my own personal war in bettering myself. In the end, look into the mirror and focus on yourself and your improvements. Some of you may never build high peaks to your biceps, or your calf development may seem nonexistent. Perhaps you are wide in the hips and less than ideal in your chest. Although the genetic framework, like that of a chassis on a car, cannot be altered, the magnificence that resides on top can always improve.

CHARTING PROGRESS

The way both this book is designed, the practitioner goes through a 12-week program that leads to a startling change. Although this idea is pretty basic, 12 weeks can often seem like a lifetime. That is why I divided the program into three 4-week phases of transformation. It's not that hard to commit to something for one lone month. Then, of course, once you see change, you will want to continue.

Your own cumulative real transformative photos will help keep the desire to change thriving. These pictures can be one of your greatest tools in obtaining your own complete physique and even for future maintenance. Pictures tell the real story: they show how you look on the outside and even offer some perspective of what's going inside—your mood and thought process. Just as pictures taken weekly will show the two main things you are looking to achieve—increased lean muscle mass and decreased fat—they are also a good check-in when going beyond the *Complete Physique* program. A picture will often tell you when it's time to floor the pedal or at least increase intensity and keep it cleaner at the dinner table.

The program has also been designed with a cheat meal built in because this is the real world we are living in. Sometimes you may miss a workout or meal here and there or even slip up. And this is okay because in between your physique goals occurs life—and sometimes life gets in the way. All I will ever ask of you is to simply give this your best shot.

In my role as personal trainer, I'm in the trenches with clients. I test ideas and make improvements to them and then record proven results and techniques here on paper for everyone to benefit from. I've never been one to change workouts just for the sake of change. I find the greatest benefit to change is simply the mental break one gets from doing the same thing over and over again. Of course *Complete Physique* offers a completely new workout, but aside from the new angles and exercises, what will always be of paramount importance is how those workouts are performed and the mental clarity and freshness that you bring week in and week out to your own program and transformation.

WHAT'S NEXT?

There are two classifications of persons: achievers and non-achievers. Some achievers do it linearly, starting at point A, then moving to point B and on to the ultimate destination, point Z. Others may start with point A, then hit Q, back up to D until ultimately arriving at Z. As this equates here, some of you will complete the 12-week program having achieved their personal best and hit all their goals. Others, not having arrived yet, will still show remarkable progress. Not everyone begins at the same starting point, and the finish line (there never really is one in the realm of health and fitness or life, for that matter) is different for everyone.

If you've made it through the *Complete Physique* program and are better in your after picture than in your before, you're an achiever. And achievers come in all shapes and sizes. So don't compare yourself to anyone. Focus on the good within you. I guarantee that the person that you look at and wonder, "If I only had what he or she has," is looking to someone else thinking the same thing.

You can still use others as inspiration, though. When I was 19 and winning my class at a national bodybuilding contest, I was coming off stage and took a gander at a competitor who was just taking to the stage. He had amazing detail in his lower body that I just didn't have. I remember wishing that I had what he had, but I was also glad we were in different weight classes. After my win, I was happy with what I had achieved: however, I did set my sights on a new goal—achieving a quality similar to that other competitor. His accomplishment hadn't stopped me or taken away the pride I felt when awarded a trophy and a title, but it did push me as you should be pushed to forever strive to improve.

So what's truly next is progressing toward your goal and letting off the throttle periodically. As long as you don't step completely off the gas and put the foot on the brake then you're still in the race. Igniting passion is easy; keeping it lit and burning through a pathway is hard. Your successful transformation will keep that passion alive.

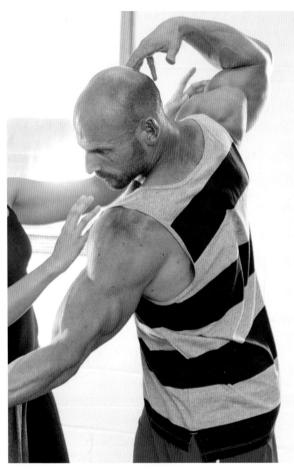

ABOUT THE MODEL

Sarah grew up less than 10 miles outside of New York City in Nutley, New Jersey. Her proximity to the theater capital of the world influenced her love of performing, and she started acting, singing and dancing at a very young age. Sarah has performed at such iconic places as Carnegie Hall and Lincoln Center. She is a proud graduate of the University of Miami with a BFA in Musical Theater. Sarah has appeared in a long list of television shows and feature films, and she is a member of the sketch group Casual Mafia. One of the web series Sarah worked in, *We Are Angels*, was an official selection of the 2012 Marseille Web Festival. Be sure to stay up to date with Sarah at www.sarahschreiber.com, or follow her on twitter @sarahschreib. For food, fitness and dog pictures, be sure to follow her on instagram @sarahschreiber

Photography

Jen Schmidt (jenschmidtphotography.com)

Art direction

Lisa Purcell

Female model

Sarah Schreiber www.sarahschreiber.com

Photographed on location at:

- Iron Fitness, Santa Monica, California, USA (ironla.com)
- Gold's Gym, Venice, California, USA (www.goldsgym.com/veniceca/)
- Fitness Factory L.A., West Hollywood, California, USA (www.fitnessfactoryla.com)

Weight belt provided by Cardillo (http://www.cardillousa.com)

Additional photography: page 7 Can Stock Photo Inc./EpicStockMedia; 15 left, 23 Championstudio; 31 left, 44 Can Stock Photo Inc./gvictoria; 31 right, 43 Can Stock Photo Inc./vanillaechoes; 41 Can Stock Photo Inc./tomboy2290; 42 Can Stock Photo Inc./Bialasiewicz; 55 Can Stock Photo Inc./expopixel; 57 Can Stock Photo Inc./4774344sean

All anatomical illustrations © Can Stock Photo Inc./Decade3D

ACKNOWLEDGMENTS

The author wishes to thank the good people of Iron Fitness, Santa Monica; Gold's Gym, Venice; Fitness Factory L.A., West Hollywood; and especially Lisa Purcell and Jen Schmidt for their tireless efforts.

ABOUT THE AUTHOR

Before his career as author and personal trainer, HOLLIS LANCE LIEBMAN has been a fitness magazine editor, national bodybuilding champion and published physique photographer, and he has also served as a bodybuilding and fitness competition judge. Hollis has worked with some of Hollywood's elite, earning himself rave reviews. *Complete Physique: Your Ultimate Body Transformation* is his third book packaged under Liebman Holdings, LLC.

Visit www.holliswashere.com to keep up with all of his things social, including fitness tips and complete training programs.

This book is dedicated to the memory of my childhood friend Mark Edward Zona. Mark grew up to become a highly intelligent and self-motivated man, fearless and highly successful in both his business and global travel pursuits. Miss you my friend. Until we meet again.